Pathology of Malignant Mesothelioma

Françoise Galateau-Sallé

Pathology of Malignant Mesothelioma

With 169 Figures, 158 in Full Color

International Mesothelioma Panel
Elisabeth Brambilla, Philip T. Cagle, Andrew M. Churg,
Thomas V. Colby, Allen R. Gibbs, Samuel P. Hammar, Philip S. Hasleton,
Douglas W. Henderson, Kouki Inai, Marleen Praet, Victor L. Roggli,
William D. Travis, Jean Michel Vignaud

Springer

Françoise Galateau-Sallé, MD
Mesopath Group, ERI3 Inserm, Laboratoire d'Anatomie Pathologique, CHU Caen, France

Special thanks to the members of the Programme National de Surveillance des Mésothéliomes supported by the Institut de Veille Sanitaire

Issam Abdalsamad[2], Hugues Begueret[2], Frederique Capron[2], Marie Christine Copin[2], AnneYvonne deLajartre[2], Armelle Foulet[2], Antoine deMascarel[2], Loulette Garbe[2], Odile Groussard[2], Jean Michel Piquenot[2], Françoise Thivolet[2], Anne deQuillacq[2], and the PNSM [Programme National de Surveillance des Mésothéliomes]; Marc Letourneux[3], Jean Claude Pairon[4,6], Patrick Rolland[5], Patrick Brochard[6], Philippe Astoul[7], Guy Launoy[8], Soizic Chamming's[6], MC Jaurand[4], Annabelle Gilg soit Ilg[5], Ellen Imbernon[5], Marcel Goldberg[5]

1. Department of Pathology CHU Caen, France
2. Mesopath Group, CHU Caen, France
3. Institut de Medecine du travail de Basse Normandie, CHU Caen France
4. INSERM E337, Creteil, France
5. Département Santé Travail, Institut de Veille Sanitaire, Saint Maurice, France
6. Isped_LSTE Bordeaux Cedex
7. Department of Respiratory Diseases, CHU Marseille, France
8. INSERM ERI 3 CHU Caen, France

British Library Cataloguing in Publication Data
A catalogue record for this book is available from the British Library

e-ISBN 1-84628-012-5
ISBN-13: 978-1-84996-939-0 e-ISBN-13: 978-1-84628-012-2

Printed on acid-free paper

Printed in China. (BS/EVB)

9 8 7 6 5 4 3 2 1

Springer Science+Business Media
springeronline.com

Preface

The Urgency of Improving and Standardizing Diagnostic Methods for Mesothelioma

Recent decades have seen substantially increased worldwide incidence and mortality rates for mesothelioma. Studies in many countries have confirmed its association with asbestos exposure. Nonetheless, important scientific and public health questions still need answers.

What morphologic and chemical characteristics of these fibers explain their carcinogenic effects? Is there a threshold below which asbestos exposure would be harmless? What risks are associated with the current conditions of occupational exposure—which are much shorter and much less intense than those observed in the historical cohorts that enabled identification of the risks associated with this material? Does spending time in buildings with asbestos have carcinogenic effects when the asbestos fibers are observed at levels substantially lower than those associated with occupational exposure? What about environmental exposures from either natural (fibers in the soil) or industrial (asbestos mines, asbestos processing plants) sources? Can asbestos induce primary pleural tumors of a histologic type other than mesothelioma? Are the man-made mineral fibers used as asbestos substitutes likely to induce mesothelioma? Are there other agents capable of such an effect? How will the mesothelioma epidemic develop in the decades to come in different countries?

Quantification of the risks associated with asbestos is also a major scientific and public health issue. Controversy surrounds the models currently used, which postulate a linear no-threshold relation, and the parameters that characterize the dose–risk curve. Risk assessments based on these models play a determinant role in forecasting incidence trends and estimating the scale of asbestos impact on populations, and they have various concrete consequences, including financial.

These questions are therefore not at all academic: They are important when determining prevention policies and financial compensation. An international mobilization of biologic, experimental, clinical, and epidemiologic research has sought to improve our understanding of these questions.

One of the most important pathways to a better understanding of all these questions involves the improvement and standardization of diagnostic methods for mesothelioma.

Scientists face many difficulties in understanding the mechanisms of this cancer's development, the role of the several varieties of asbestos and of a wide range of other factors, and the extent of the consequences of asbestos exposure. More problems come when interpreting past incidence trends and when forecasting future trends. Many of these issues are related to limitations in our capacity to diagnose mesothelioma and in the difficulty pathologists face in finding methods that are sensitive, specific, and reproducible from an international perspective. The subsequent failure to identify cases and the inaccurate diagnoses of metastases and other forms of pleura-based tumors such as mesotheliomas cause individual harm; bias epidemiologic surveys, mesothelioma incidence estimates, and international comparisons; and impede the study of changes in this cancer's incidence over time. These factors have led to important scientific (and legal) debates in a variety of circumstances.

Publication of this work by the International Mesothelioma Panel is therefore particularly welcome. It provides information about recent advances—some quite spectacular—in methods for diagnosing mesothelioma. Let us hope that this volume will promote diffusion of the most effective of these methods to the vast number of pathologists who are not specialized in this domain but who must occasionally examine this tumor.

Mesothelioma is still a complex scientific and public health problem, and all the forecasts indicate that it will remain with us for at least several more decades. Constant improvement of diagnostic methods is urgently needed to improve our understanding and management of it. Future work by the International Mesothelioma Panel to improve early detection through the new tools now available to pathologists (e.g., molecular biology, immunohistochemistry) will help with the international resolution of this question, a resolution today still in its first stages.

Marcel Goldberg
INSERM Unit 88
Epidemiology, Public Health and Occupational and General Environment
Hôpital National de Saint-Maurice
14, rue du Val d'Osne
94415 Saint-Maurice Cedex, France

Acknowledgments

To Sofia, Eva, Eloïse, Alix, Pierre, Iris, and Nathan

To Guillaume and Maria, Ariane and Thomas, Yan and Karine, Stéphane and Caroline for the time I spent not being with them, to my husband, to my parents and to my family for their loving support and understanding during my work on this book.

I am particularly grateful to my contributors for their great assistance toward the completion of this monograph and also grateful for their trust in me, their insightful comments that have enhanced my understanding of mesothelioma, and the great pleasure they gave me working in their company.

Thanks to Ariane Galateau for her great photographic assistance.

Thanks to Gilles Anquetil, photographer for his great technical assistance to CHU CAEN and to Conseil Regional de Basse Normandie. This work was supported in part by funds from the Ministère de l'Emploi et de la Solidarité (DGS, DRT), Paris, France.

I dedicate this book to our readers, hoping they will find in this monograph assistance and answers to their questions.

Contents

Contributor List

Members of the International Mesothelioma Panel

Panel Chair:

Françoise Galateau-Sallé, MD
Mesopath Group / INSERM ERI 3, Laboratoire d'Anatomie Pathologique, CHU Caen, France

Panel Members:

Professor Elisabeth Brambilla, MD, PhD
Laboratoire de Pathologie Cellulaire, INSERM U578, CHU Grenoble, France

Philip T. Cagle, MD
Department of Pathology, Center for Pulmonary Pathology, Baylor College of Medicine, Houston, TX, USA

Andrew M. Churg, MD, PhD
Department of Pathology, University of British Columbia, School of Medicine, Vancouver, BC, Canada

Thomas V. Colby, MD
Department of Pathology and Laboratory Science, Mayo Clinic Scottsdale Scottsdale, AZ, USA

Allen R. Gibbs, MB ChB, FRCPath
Department of Histopathology, Llandough Hospital, Cardiff and Vale NHS Trust Penarth, UK

Samuel P. Hammar, MD
Diagnostic Specialties Laboratory, Bremerton, WA, USA

Philip S. Hasleton, MD, FRCPath
Department of Pulmonary Pathology, Manchester University, UK

Douglas W. Henderson, MBBS, FRCPA, FRCPath, FHKCPath
Department of Anatomical Pathology, Flinders Medical Centre, Bedford Park, SA, Australia

Kouki Inai, MD, PhD
Department of Pathology, Graduate School of Biomedical Sciences, Hiroshima University, Japan

Marleen Praet, MD, PhD
University Hospital Department of Pathology, N. Goormachtigh Institute for Pathology, Faculty of Medicine and Health Sciences, Ghent University, Belgium

Victor L. Roggli, MD
Department of Pathology, Duke University and Durham VA Medical Centers, Durham, NC, USA

William D. Travis, MD
Department of Pulmonary and Mediastinal Pathology, Armed Forces Institute of Pathology, Washington, DC, USA

Jean Michel Vignaud, MD
Laboratoire d'Anatomie Pathologique, INSERM EMI 14 CHU de Nancy, France

With collaboration of

Alain Jehan, MD
Service de Pneumologie, CHU Caen Cote de Nacre, France

Philippe Astoul, MD
Departement des maladies respiratoires_unité d'oncologie
Marseille, France

1
Epidemiology of Mesothelioma

Malignant mesothelioma has risen from obscurity and rarity during the first half of the twentieth century to become a major occupational and public health problem late in the latter half of that century and the beginning of the twenty-first century. The nexus between asbestos exposure and subsequent development of mesothelioma was established definitively in 1960 by Wagner et al. [1] in South Africa. By the late 1990s, the incidence of mesothelioma in some industrialized nations was roughly comparable to that of cancer of the larynx [2], and the mortality rate was similar to that for renal cell carcinoma in men and for uterine cancer in women [2–4]. Apart from lung cancer, mesothelioma constitutes the most important occupational cancer among industrial workers.

Most mesotheliomas encountered during the early twenty-first century are a consequence of prior occupational exposure to asbestos from the 1940s through the 1970s, including end-use and bystander exposures [5, 6]. The relation between inhalation of asbestos fibers—especially one or more of the amphibole varieties—and mesothelioma is accepted by almost all authorities as causal; because of the consistency and specificity of the asbestos-mesothelioma relation, the incidence of mesothelioma is usually considered to be an index of societies' past usage of asbestos (Table 1.1) [7–10].

Recent incidence rates for mesothelioma in various countries are listed in Table 1.1 and are generally in the range of 14 to 30 cases per million persons per year (>15 years of age) [9, 10]. The highest incidence is found in Australia, where the rate in 1997 was 29.8/million persons/year (50.6/million/year for males and 9.0/million/year for females, standardized to the world population >20 years of age, whereas the corresponding crude rates in 1997 for Australia were 59.8/million for males and 10.9/million for females) [4]. In the United States, the current rate for the sexes combined is 10.0/million/year [11].

It has been estimated that about 10,000 mesotheliomas occur annually throughout North America, Australia, and seven nations in western Europe and Scandinavia [9]. Peto et al. [5] predicted about 190,000 mesothelioma

TABLE 1.1. Mesothelioma incidence across nations relative to historical use of asbestos*

Nation	Mesothelioma incidence (cases/million/year)	Use of asbestos (kg/capita/year)
Australia (1995)	33	4.4 (1968)
The Netherlands (1995)	27	3.4 (1976)
United Kingdom (1991)	23	2.7 (1970)
Italy (1993)	22	2.5 (1975)
France (1996)	17	2.6 (1970)
Finland (1995)	15	2.2 (1970)
Germany (1997)	15	3.0 (1975)
Sweden (1995)	15	2.4 (1970)
United States (1999)	10	2.3 (1975)
Norway (1995)	14	1.9 (1970)

Modified from Tossavainen [9].

deaths across six nations in western Europe (Britain, France, Germany, Italy, The Netherlands, and Switzerland) over the 35-year period dating from 1999. Modeling of data for France indicates that mortality from mesothelioma among French men aged 50 to 79 will continue to increase, reaching a peak of 1140 deaths in 2030 (optimistic forecast) to 1300 deaths in 2040 (pessimistic prediction), and no preventive measures implemented at this time can affect this trend [12]. In Australia, the incidence of mesothelioma is expected to peak in about 2020 (approximately 18,000 cases for the period 1945–2020) [4]. In the United States, the peak incidence was predicted to occur by the year 2000, with a slow decline thereafter [7]. In the United Kingdom, the rate of increase in mesothelioma-related deaths slowed slightly in 1997, when there were 1330 deaths, but the rate increased thereafter, with 1535 deaths in 1998 and 1595 in 1999 [13]; the crude death rate for mesothelioma in Great Britain rose from 29.57 per million for males during 1989–1991 to 40.93 during 1995–1997, and for the same periods the equivalent death rate in females rose from 4.67 to 5.77 [14]. The Health and Safety Executive [15] estimated that deaths from mesothelioma in men in the United Kingdom "may peak around the year 2011, at about 1700 deaths per year," whereas mesothelioma-related deaths in women "are running at about one-sixth of the level in men." In this respect, mesothelioma incidence rates have increased about fourfold or fivefold in Australia over a period of almost 20 years, and the rate in females has also increased about threefold; however, the male incidence is more than five times that in females [4]. In some nations, the time trend of increasing incidence after 1986 is restricted largely to those aged over 50 years, suggesting that controls on occupational exposures introduced from the 1970s have been effective [4]. However, this is not the case for all industrialized countries. In France, for instance, the relative risk of developing a pleural mesothelioma among men is 1.83 for the youngest generation (men born in 1953) compared to the 1928 generation [16], whereas the maximum risk for males occurs for the 1925–1929 birth cohort in the United States [17]. These contrasting findings show that awareness about the danger of asbestos exposure effects was not the same in all countries.

Asbestos Exposure and Mesothelioma

In national registries, about 90% of male mesothelioma patients have a history of asbestos exposure, especially those with pleural mesotheliomas, with a somewhat smaller percentage for patients with peritoneal mesothelioma (about 60%) [4, 18]. The proportion of asbestos-associated mesotheliomas is lower in females and varies among countries, ranging from 25% in the United States to as much as 70% in Australia [4, 18]. In some series a small number of the exposures are occupational, so nonoccupational exposures comprise a much larger proportion of mesothelioma cases among women [19]. Roggli et al. [19] found that the lung tissue asbestos burden was elevated in 70% of a series of female mesothelioma patients in the United States: the main fiber type was amosite, followed by tremolite.

The occupations producing the greatest number of mesotheliomas have changed over the years from miners/millers and those involved in product manufacture and insulation work to other end-users of asbestos-containing products, most notably persons in building construction and demolition industries and in shipyards [6–8, 13, 20], in part because working conditions in the building industry in particular have been poorly regulated. Individual life-time risks of mesothelioma are highest among crocidolite miners/millers, power station workers, railways laborers, and naval, merchant naval, and shipyard personnel [4]. However, the number of personnel employed in each of the last-cited occupations are smaller than in the building construction industry, so carpenters/joiners, for example, contribute greater absolute numbers to national mesothelioma tolls, although the individual risk is less [4]. Substantial numbers of mesotheliomas are now seen as a consequence of nonoccupational exposures, including occasional "handyman"-type exposure, domestic exposure (e.g., from laundering asbestos-contaminated work clothes), and other types of occasional or non-occupational exposures [4, 6, 21, 22]. Mesothelioma has been reported to occur after brief low-level or indirect exposure [23].

The risk or incidence of mesothelioma shows a dose-response relation to cumulative asbestos exposure, so the risk is greatest with heavy exposures [24, 25], and peritoneal mesotheliomas [26] are usually related to heavier cumulative exposures than pleural mesotheliomas. In general, the incidence of mesothelioma in asbestos-exposed cohorts reflects the fiber type or types, cumulative exposure, and the time following exposure so remote exposures are more significant for mesothelioma induction than recent exposures, other factors being equal [24].

Asbestos occurs in two major mineralogic groups: the amphiboles (of which amosite and crocidolite constitute the major commercial forms) and chrysotile [27]. Over recent decades, chrysotile comprised about 95% of world asbestos production, most originating from Canada and Russia [6]. Fibrous tremolite, anthophyllite, and actinolite constitute other forms of amphibole asbestos. Production of these minerals, however, was restricted to only a few mines or industries, although small amounts of fibrous tremolite occur in Canadian chrysotile (usually about 1% or less), and tremolite was used in certain regions (e.g., as a whitewash in Greece and Cyprus and in New Caledonia) [6]. Although it has been claimed that all varieties of commercial asbestos have the capacity for mesothelioma induction, there is general agreement that crocidolite is the most potent type of asbestos for mesothelioma induction, followed by amosite and then chrysotile [6, 28]. There is much debate regarding the ability of chrysotile to cause mesothelioma. Some of the differences relate to interpretation of the epidemiologic data, but at the heart of the controversy lie the differing views on the importance of biopersistence in carcinogenesis and the significance of chrysotile contamination by tremolite. The association between mesothelioma and chrysotile exposure is largely based on studies of the Quebec chrysotile miners and millers, a situation where tremolite contamination of the chrysotile ore is well recognized [29, 30]. It is outside the scope of this volume to debate this issue, and the reader is referred elsewhere [28–38]. The greater potency of the amphiboles for mesothelioma induction compared to that of chrysotile is thought to be related to the fiber characteristics and to the greater biopersistence of amphibole fibers in lung tissue than chrysotile (which fragments or dissolves more rapidly), so the half-life of chrysotile (weeks to months) in lung parenchyma is much shorter than the half-life for the amphiboles (years to decades) [6, 38]. The factors influencing fiber clearance from the lung were well summarized by Roggli and Brody [39].

Fiber dimensions are also thought to be important for mesothelioma induction, so short-length fibers have little carcinogenic activity in comparison to long-length fibers (>5 μm in length and especially >8–10 μm in length) [6, 40]. Boutin et al. [41] demonstrated asbestos fibers concentrated in parietal pleural "black spots" in exposed subjects. Amphiboles outnumbered chrysotile in all samples: 22.5% of fibers were 5 μm or longer in the black spots. The black spots were histologically similar to milky spots as seen by conventional and electron microscopy. These findings may well explain why the parietal pleura is the target organ for mesothelioma and plaques.

Most mesotheliomas now encountered among the populations of Europe, North America, and Australaia occur in individuals with a history of mixed asbestos inhalation (e.g., chrysotile plus amosite fibers released by operations on insulation materials or high-density asbestos-cement building products) [6].

It should be remembered that a history of exposure to asbestos or the lack thereof is important when assigning causation to a malignant mesothelioma. However, a history of exposure to asbestos should play no role in the diagnosis; diagnosis depends on the gross, microscopic and special-technique observations, as it does with any other tumor.

Latency

There is characteristically a prolonged time interval (i.e., latency) between the first inhalation of asbestos and the subsequent diagnosis of mesothelioma, generally in the range of 20 to 40 years [37]. For most mesotheliomas, the latency is more than 20 years, with 15 years or less for only about 1% of mesotheliomas [13, 42–44]; some authorities delineate a minimum lag-time of 15 years from exposure and others 10 years [43]. When the latency is less than 10 to 15 years, it is likely that the proximate exposure was coincidental and that there were one or more unrecognized exposures more remote in time [38].

Other Factors Implicated in the Induction of Mesothelioma

Despite strong association with past asbestos exposure, there are other mesotheliomas for which the cause is unknown [45].

Erionite is a naturally occurring fibrous zeolite and is known to induce mesothelioma among the inhabitants of certain villages in the Cappadocian region of Turkey [46–48]. Erionite has fiber dimensions and properties similar to those of amphibole forms of asbestos.

There are anecdotal reports of mesothelioma following *irradiation*, including radiotherapy for childhood cancers such as Wilms' tumor; cases of mesothelioma have also been reported following injection of radioactive thorium dioxide (Thorotrast) for radiologic investigations (for references, see elsewhere [22–49]). However, a retrospective cohort study on a large group of women with breast cancer and patients with Hodgkin's disease—many of whom had been treated by radiotherapy—found no significant increase in the relative risk of mesothelioma [50]. In addition, coexisting asbestos exposure represents a confounding factor for some cases associated with irradiation: In one report on mortality among plutonium workers, all the mesotheliomas occurred in patients who had also sustained asbestos exposure [51]. The incidence of mesothelioma was not increased (as a second malignancy) in one study of patients with prior radiation therapy [52].

Prior Inflammatory Disorders Affecting Serosal Membranes

Mesotheliomas have occurred years after chronic inflammatory lesions of the pleura (e.g., chronic empyema or packing of the pleural cavity with lucite spheres as treatment for tuberculosis (plombage therapy)), and there are a few reports (about eight 8 cases) of an association with familial Mediterranean fever (FMF), possibly related to recurrent FMF serositis [53]. However, cases of this type are exceptional. For example, in relation to FMF, cases of mesothelioma have been reported in the Mediterranean region after white-washing homes with tremolite-containing material [54,55]. Most cases of "postinflammatory" mesothelioma with a short interval between inflammation and tumor are probably mesotheliomas that presented with a burst of inflammatory activity followed by a period of quiescence [56].

Simian Virus 40 and Mesothelioma

A voluminous literature has grown rapidly on the detection of simian virus 40 (SV40) DNA in up to 60% of human mesotheliomas (see Chapter 2). These reports followed an initial observation that SV40 induces mesothelioma in experimental animals when injected into the pleural cavity [57]. For humans, early poliomyelitis vaccines contaminated with SV40 were a potential source for the SV40 DNA. However, the evidence in favor of SV40 as a cofactor for mesothelioma induction is still inconclusive, and a recent position statement from the British Thoracic Society evaluated the evidence for this relation as "weak" [58].

Familial Factors

The clustering of mesothelioma within families has been reported in several articles, which has suggested a genetic susceptibility to the tumor [59]. Some have occurred in the apparent absence of asbestos exposure, whereas others have also been associated with asbestos exposure. However, the genetic and biologic differences between asbestos-related and non-asbestos-related tumors are unclear [60]. A recent report described a family of three sisters who developed mesothelioma in association with environmental-residential exposure to asbestos; in two of the cases, comparative genomic hybridization showed a loss only at 9p; and it was suggested that this region might be a site of one or more oncosuppressor genes, which might be related to increased genetic susceptibility to the carcinogenetic effects of asbestos [61].

References

1. Wagner JC, Sleggs CA, Marchand P. Diffuse pleural mesothelioma and asbestos exposure in the North Western Cape Province. Br J Ind Med 1960;17:260–71.

2. South Australian Cancer Registry. Epidemiology of cancer in South Australia: incidence, mortality and survival 1977 to 1999. Adelaide: Department of Human Services; 2000.
3. New South Wales Cancer Council (NSWCC). Cancer in New South Wales: incidence and mortality 1997. Sydney: NSWCC; 1999.
4. Leigh J, Davidson P, Hendrie L, Berry D. Malignant mesothelioma in Australia, 1945–2000. J Occup Health Safety Aust NZ 2001;17:453–70.
5. Peto J, Decarli A, La Vecchia C, et al. The European mesothelioma epidemic. Br J Cancer 1999;79:666–72.
6. World Trade Organization (WTO): European Communities—measures concerning asbestos and asbestos-containing products. Geneva: WTO; 2000 (www.wto.org).
7. Price B. Analysis of current trends in United States mesothelioma incidence. Am J Epidemiol 1997;145:211–18.
8. Teschke K, Morgan MS, Checkoway H, et al. Mesothelioma surveillance to locate sources of exposure to asbestos. Can J Public Health 1997;88:163–8.
9. Tossavainen A. Asbestos, asbestosis and cancer: exposure criteria for clinical diagnosis. In: People and Work Research Reports, vol 14. Helsinki: Finnish Institute of Occupational Health 1997;14:8–27.
10. Tossavainen A, Takahashi K. Epidemiological trends for asbestos-related cancers. In: People and Work Research Reports, vol 36. Helsinki: Finnish Institute of Occupational Health 2000;36:26–30.
11. Price B, Ware A. Mesothelioma trends in the United States: an update based on Surveillance, Epidemiology, and End Results Program data for 1973 through 2003. Am J Epidemiol 2004;159:107–12.
12. Banaei A, Auvert B, Goldberg M, et al. Future trends in mortality of French men from mesothelioma. Occup Environ Med 2000;57:488–94.
13. Health & Safety Executive (HSE). Health and safety statistics 2000/01. London: HSE Books; 2001 (http://www.hse.gov.uk/statistics/2001/hsspt2.pdf).
14. HSE. Health and Safety Statistics 1998/99. London: HSE Books; 1999.
15. Health and Safety Executive. Mesothelioma Occupation Statistics: male and female deaths aged 16–74 in Great Britain: 1980–2000 (excluding 1981). Available on the HSE website 2003.
16. Remontet L, Esteve J, Bouvier AM, et al. Cancer incidence and mortality in France over the period 1978–2000. Rev Epidemiol Sante Publique 2003;51: 3–30.
17. Harris LV, Kahwa IA. Asbestos: old foe in 21st century developing countries. Sci Total Environ 2003;307:1–3.
18. Spirtas R, Heineman EF, Bernstein L, et al. Malignant mesothelioma: attributable risk of asbestos exposure. Occup Environ Med 1994;51:804–11.
19. Roggli VL, Oury TD, Moffatt EJ. Malignant mesothelioma in women. Anat Pathol 1997;2:147–63.
20. Albin M, Magnani C, Krstev S, et al. Asbestos and cancer: an overview of current trends in Europe. Environ Health Perspect 1999;107(Suppl 2):289–98.
21. Schneider J, Woitowitz H-J. Asbestos-related non-occupational malignant mesothelioma. In: Peters GA, Peters BJ (eds) Sourcebook on asbestos diseases, vol 17. Charlottesville, VA: Lexis; 1998;43–69.
22. Hillerdal G. Mesothelioma: cases associated with non-occupational and low dose exposures. Occup Environ Med 1999;56:505–13.

23. Iwatsubo Y, Pairon JC, Boutin C, et al. Pleural mesothelioma: dose-response relation at low levels of asbestos exposure in a French population-based case-control study. Am J Epidemiol 1998;148:133–42.
24. De Klerk NH, Armstrong BK. The epidemiology of asbestos and mesothelioma. In: Henderson DW, Shilkin KB, Langlois SL, Whitaker D (eds) Malignant mesothelioma. New York: Hemisphere; 1992:223–50.
25. Berry G, Newhouse ML, Wagner JC. Mortality from all cancers of asbestos factory workers in east London 1933–80. Occup Environ Med 2000;57: 782–5.
26. Neumann V, Muller KM, Fischer M. Peritoneal mesothelioma—incidence and etiology. Pathologie 1999;20:169–76.
27. Roggli VL, Coin P. Mineralogy of asbestos. In: Roggli VL, Greenberg SD, Pratt PC (eds) Pathology of asbestos-associated diseases. Boston: Little, Brown; 1992:1–17.
28. Hodgson JT, Darnton A. The quantitative risks of mesothelioma and lung cancer in relation to asbestos exposure. Ann Occup Hyg 2000;44:565–601.
29. McDonald JC, McDonald AD. Chrysotile, tremolite and carcinogenicity. Ann Occup Hyg 1997;91:699–705.
30. McDonald, C. Asbestos in epidemiology of work related diseases, 2nd edition. London: BMJ Publishing Group; 2000:102–3.
31. Mossman BT, Gee JB. Asbestos-related cancer and the amphibole hypothesis. Am J Public Health 1997;87:689–90.
32. Cullen MR. Chrysotile asbestos: enough is enough. Lancet 1998;351:1377–8.
33. Stayner LT, Dankovic DA, Lemen RA. Occupational exposure to chrysotile asbestos and cancer risk: a review of the amphibole hypothesis. Am J Public Health 1996;86;179–86.
34. McDonald JC, McDonald AD. Asbestos and carcinogenicity. Science 1990; 249:844.
35. Stanton MF, Layard M, Tegeris, et al. Relation of particle dimension to carcinogenicity in amphibole asbestoses and other fibrous minerals. J Natl Cancer Inst 1981;67:965–75.
36. Wagner JC. Asbestos-related cancer and the amphibole hypothesis. Am J Public Health 1997;87:487–8.
37. Berman DW, Crump KS. Final draft: technical support document for a protocol to assess asbestos-related risk. Washington, DC: U.S. Environmental Protection Agency, 2004.
38. Churg A. Neoplastic asbestos-induced disease. In: Churg A, Green FHY (eds) Pathology of occupational lung disease, 2nd edition. Baltimore: Williams & Wilkins; 1998:339–91.
39. Roggli, VL, Brody, AR. Experimental models of asbestos-related diseases. In: Roggli VL, Greenberg SD, Pratt PC (eds) Pathology of asbestos-associated diseases. Boston: Little, Brown; 1992:257–97.
40. Report of the expert panel on health effects of asbestos and synthetic vitreous fibers: the influence of fiber length. Washington, DC: Agency for Toxic Substances and Disease Registry, U.S. Department of Health and Human Services, 2003.
41. Boutin C, Dumortier P, Rey F, et al. Black spots concentrate oncogenic asbestos fibers in the parietal pleura: thoracoscopic and mineralogic study. Am J Respir Crit Care Med 1996;153:444–9.

42. Ferguson DA, Berry G, Jelihovsky T, et al. The Australian mesothelioma surveillance program 1979–1985. Med J Aust 1987;147:166–72.
43. Lanphear BP, Buncher CR. Latent period for malignant mesothelioma of occupational origin. J Occup Med 1992;34:718–21.
44. Woitowitz H-J, Kraus T. Screening of asbestos-exposed workers in Germany. In: People and Work Research Reports, vol 36. Helsinki: Finnish Institute of Occupational Health; 2000:42–52.
45. McDonald JC, McDonald AD. Mesothelioma: is there a background? In: Jaurand M-C, Bignon J (eds) The mesothelial cell and mesothelioma. New York: Marcel Dekker; 1994:37–45.
46. Baris I, Simonato L, Artvinli M, et al. Epidemiological and environmental evidence of the health effects of exposure to erionite fibers: a four-year study in the Cappadocian region of Turkey. Int J Cancer 1987;39:10–17.
47. Baris YI, Simonato L, Saracci R, et al. The epidemic of respiratory cancer associated with erionite fibers in the Cappadocian region of Turkey. In: Elliott P, Cuzick J, English D, (eds) Geographical and environmental epidemiology: methods for small-area studies. Oxford: Oxford University Press; 1992: 310–22.
48. Metintas M, Hillerdal G, Metintas S. Malignant mesothelioma due to environmental exposure to erionite: follow-up of a Turkish emigrant cohort. Eur Respir J 1999;13:523–6.
49. Comin CE, de Klerk NH, Henderson DW. Malignant mesothelioma: current conundrums over risk estimates, and whither electron microscopy for diagnosis? Ultrastruct Pathol 1997;21:315–20.
50. Neugut AI, Ahsan H, Antman KH. Incidence of malignant pleural mesothelioma after thoracic radiotherapy. Cancer 1997;80:948–50.
51. Gold B, Kathren RL. Causes of death in a cohort of 260 plutonium workers. Health Phys 1998;75:236–40.
52. Cavazza LB, Travis WD, Travis JT III, et al. Post-irradiation malignant mesothelioma. Cancer 1996;77:1379–85.
53. Gentiloni N, Febbraro S, Barone C, et al. Peritoneal mesothelioma in recurrent familial peritonitis. J Clin Gastroenterol 1997;24:276–9.
54. Sakellariou K, Malamou-Mitsi V, Haritou A, et al. Malignant pleural mesothelioma from nonoccupational asbestos exposure in Metsovo (north-west Greece): slow end of an epidemic? Eur Respir J 1996;9:1206–10.
55. Constantopoulos SH, Sakellariou K. Non-occupational mesothelioma: epidemiological considerations. In: Peters GA, Peters BJ (eds) Sourcebook on asbestos diseases, vol 17. Charlottesville: VA: Lexis; 1998;17:71–97.
56. Henderson DW, Comin CE, Hammar SP, et al. Malignant mesothelioma of the pleura: current surgical pathology. In: Corrin B (ed) Pathology of lung tumors. New York: Churchill Livingstone; 1997:241–80.
57. Cicala C, Pompetti F, Carbone M. SV40 induces mesotheliomas in hamsters. Am J Pathol 1993;142:1524–33.
58. Statement on malignant mesothelioma in the United Kingdom: British Thoracic Society Standards of Care Committee. Thorax 2001;56:250–65.
59. Dawson A, Gibbs AR, Browne K, et al. Familial mesothelioma: details of 17 cases with hitopathologic findings and mineral analysis. Cancer 1992;70:1183–7.
60. Huncharek M. Non-asbestos related diffuse malignant mesothelioma. Tumori 2002;88:1–9.

61. Musti M, Cavone D, Aalto Y, et al. A cluster of familial malignant mesothelioma with del(9p) as sole chromosomal abnormality. Cancer Genet Cytogenet 2002; 138:73–6.

2
Molecular Biology

The 20- to 40-year latency for the development of mesothelioma suggests that multiple genetic alterations are required for tumorigenic conversion of a normal to a malignant mesothelial cell. Although the lung fiber burden depends on the particular fiber type and the extent of exposure [1], the biopersistence of the more carcinogenic amphibole fibers is significantly higher than that of the serpentine-type fibers, as shown by rat lung inhalation studies [2, 3]. The long latency from the time of initial asbestos exposure to diagnosis [4] and the early recognition of recurrent chromosomal abnormalities in malignant mesothelioma provide early support for multiple clonal chromosomal abnormalities and multistep carcinogenesis in the development of mesothelioma. This chapter reviews the mechanisms of asbestos-induced oncogenesis, the abnormal expression of oncogenes and growth factors induced by fibers, the chromosomal damage induced by asbestos and observed in malignant mesothelioma including chromosomal deletion and chromosomal polysomy, both reflecting genomic instability, and the role of well identified tumor suppressor genes such as $p16^{\mathrm{INK4}}$, *p53*, and *NF2* and of two mechanisms of inactivation of tumor suppressor genes, MDM2 and SV40, in malignant mesothelioma.

Mechanisms of Asbestos-induced Oncogenesis

There are presently several indications that asbestos may act directly at a mitotic level and indirectly via induction of reactive oxygen and nitrogen species and growth factors. Experimental evidence shows asbestos in tissue culture can interfere with normal chromosomal segregation (mis-segregation of chromosomes) by interacting with the mitotic apparatus, leading to aneuploidy [5]. In vitro experiments have also shown that human mesothelial cells acquire extensive numerical and structural chromosomal abnormalities shortly after exposure to a low concentration of asbestos fibers [6]. Some of the most frequent numerical changes observed in vitro are identical to those commonly reported in malignant mesothelioma. These changes induce loss of one copy of chromosome 22, which is strongly associated in human malignant mesothelioma with a mutation of the resting allele.

Molecular Targets of Asbestos-induced Reactive Oxygen and Nitrogen Species

The molecular targets of asbestos and its second messengers, reactive oxygen species (ROS) and reactive nitrogen species (RNS), include critical biologic macromolecules such as lipid membranes, DNA, and signal transduction proteins. Iron compounds linked to asbestos are involved in lipid peroxidation, which modifies membrane structure and function [7, 8]. Asbestos also causes cellular toxicity by damaging DNA in cell-free systems in both pulmonary epithelial cells and pleural mesothelial cells: It causes altered DNA bases, DNA single-strand breaks [8], chromosomal alterations, and sister chromatid exchanges. DNA basepair alterations are probably caused by iron derived hydroxyl radicals (OH^-) [9]. Asbestos fibers, unlike nonfibrogenic particules, induce apoptosis in normal mesothelial cells. However, mesothelioma cell lines are highly resistant to asbestos or OH-induced apoptosis. The resistance to apoptosis in malignant mesothelioma compared to that of normal mesothelial cells is still unclear. It is not linked to disruption of the Bcl2 and bax equilibrium [10], which can modulate the susceptibility of cells to apoptosis. In the absence of Bcl2 expression, increased activity of antioxidant defenses essentially due to manganese superoxide dismutase [11] and catalase may account for the resistance of malignant mesothelial cells to oxidant-induced apoptosis.

Reactive oxygen species and asbestos-induced DNA damage stimulate a signal transduction cascade. Asbestos can activate MAP-kinase signaling pathways through the epithelial growth factor (EGF) receptor. Several of the transcription factors induced in this pathway, such as NFκB, AP1 (C-fos, C-Jun), and C-myc, are found highly expressed in mesothelioma. Most of these cytokines, growth factors, adhesion molecules, nitrogen oxygen species (NOS), and C-myc are regulated by NFκB transcription factor. AP1 transcription factors (C-fos and C-Jun) participate in inflammation and fibrotic and proliferative responses to fibers. ROS induces early genes C-*fos* and C-*myc*. How the balance between apoptosis and proliferation is skewed toward proliferation and the loss of apoptosis in malignant mesothelioma is still unclear. Further investigations are necessary to determine the factors regulating the balance between ROS and asbestos-induced DNA damage that stimulates proliferation signals and mutagenesis in contrast to those triggering cell death in normal mesothelial cells.

Abnormal Expression of Oncogenes and Growth Factors

Autocrine activity for platelet-derived growth factor (PDGF), transforming growth factor-β (TGFβ1 and TGFβ2) and EGF has been detected in conditioned media of mesothelioma cell lines [12]. Overexpression of PDGF protein and PDGF receptors has been reported, suggesting an autocrine loop of growth in mesothelioma [13, 14]. Results are, however, conflicting at the moment. Although normal mesothelial cells express both α and β receptors of PDGF A and B chains, mesotheliomas often produce PDGF A-chain and B-chain and α-receptors but not β-receptors. It is thought that PDGF A-chain maintains an autocrine loop of growth through the α-receptor. Antisense oligonucleotides against PDGF A-chain inhibit growth of some mesothelioma cell lines, whereas antisense oligonucleotides against PDGF B-chain do not. Other growth factors and cytokines are produced at high levels in mesothelioma cells, such as TGF-α, insulin-derived growth factor-1 (IGF-1), interleukin-1α (IL-1α), IL-1β, granulocyte and granulocyte/macrophage colony-stimulating factors (G-CSF, GM-CSF), monocyte chemotactic protein (MCP-1), leukocyte inhibiting factor (LIF), tumor necrosis factor-α (TNFα), IL-6, and IL-8 [15–16].

Cytogenetic Abnormalities in Malignant Mesothelioma

Karyotypic analysis has shown that malignant mesotheliomas display multiple clonal chromosomal abnormalities [17–19]. Most mesotheliomas display more than 10 clonal chromosomal abnormalities [19]. Specific deletion of chromosomal sites involves the short arm (p) of chromosomes 1, 3, and 9 and the long arm (q) of chromosome 6. The most frequent genetic change is the loss of one entire copy of chromosome 22. These are the "hot spots" of chromosomal deletion sites. In addition, malignant mesothelioma includes nonrandom cytogenic alterations on chromosomes 4, 6, 14, 15, 18, and 19 and trisomies and polysomies of chromosomes 1, 5, 7, 11, 12, and 20. Most of these cytogenetic abnormalities are found in combination in any given malignant mesothelioma, all of them being present in about 25% of malignant mesotheliomas [20]. This pattern is consistent with a multistep pathogenetic process.

Comparative genomic hybridization (CGH analysis), which is based on measuring DNA chromosomal imbalance, has shown that malignant mesothelioma exhibits multiple genomic imbalances [21]. Data from CGH are consistent with those provided earlier by karyotypic analysis, which have shown the underrepresentation of chromosome 22q in 50% of cases, loss of material at chromosomes 1p, 6q, and 9p in 40% of cases each, and loss of 3p in one-third of cases. In addition, about 50% of cases show losses at 15q11.1–q21, 42% at 14q24.2-qter, and 42% at 13q12–q14.

Statistically significant correlations have been found between a high content of asbestos fibers in lung tissue from mesothelioma patients and partial or total losses of chromosomes 1 and 4 as well as a breakpoint at locus 1p11–p22 ($p = 0.0001$, $p = 0.003$, and $p = 0.009$, respectively). This confirms the direct role of the asbestos burden in mesothelial mutagenesis. In addition, an increased copy number of chromosome 7, reflecting genetic instability, is inversely correlated with survival ($p = 0.02$) [22].

Loss of heterozygosity (LOH) analysis has allowed specific localization of tumor suppressor genes. At chromosome 1p the shortest regions of overlap of losses examined pointed to 1p21–22 representing a 4cM segment currently undergoing testing for potential tumor suppressor gene mapping. Allelic loss of 1p21–22 occurs in more than 70% of mesotheliomas [23].

The most frequent allelic deletion on chromosome 3p occurs at 3p21.3 (70%), which is also a site of frequent allelic deletion in lung carcinoma. Several candidate suppressor genes are being sought in this region, including semaphorins 3F and 3A, β-catenin, and RAS SF1.

Deletions at multiple sites on chromosome 4 are frequent in malignant mesothelioma [24]. Both cytogenetic and CGH studies have suggested that chromosome 4 deletions are involved in the pathogenesis of malignant mesothelioma. LOH studies using polymorphic probes at this region indicated that region 1 (4q33–34), region 2 (4q25–26), and region 4 (4p15.1–15.3) are sites of frequent losses (80%, 60%, and 50%, respectively) in malignant mesothelioma, which suggests that at least three candidate tumor suppressor genes should be sought in these regions.

Allelic loss at 6q occurs in 61% of malignant mesotheliomas [25]. Deletion mapping identified four specific regions—6q14–q21, 6q16.6–q21, 6q21–q23.2, and 6q25—which are also found in other malignancies, including breast cancer, ovarian cancer, and non-Hodgkin's lymphoma. Microcell-mediated chromosome transfer using three 6q regions (6q14–21, 6q21–23, 6q26–27) have independently caused reversion of tumor phenotypes in ovarian and breast cancer [26–28]. Active search for tumor suppressor genes in these regions is under way.

Fifty percent loss of chromosome 15q11.1 q21 was detected by CGH analysis [21]. The minimum region of overlap of chromosomal loss in mesotheliomas is 15q11.1–15. Interestingly, RAD51 located at 15q15.1 is potentially a relevant gene acting as a tumor suppressor gene. The RAD51 product participates in the repair of double-strand DNA breaks in chromosomal dysjunction, and mutation of the mouse RAD51 has been associated with severe chromosomal loss in actively dividing cells [29]. The 13q12–14 site of recurrent loss in mesothelioma (42%) is the location of the *BRCA2* gene, whose product is an essential cofactor of RAD51-dependent DNA repair of double-strand breaks [30].

Chromosome 9p21 is a region homozygously deleted in 85% of malignant mesothelioma cell lines and 22% of primary malignant mesotheliomas [31]. $P16^{INK4A}$ but not $P15^{INK4B}$ is deleted [32]. The shortest region of overlap of this homozygous deletion is a 1-megabase segment situated distal to the interferon gene cluster that contains two tumor suppressor genes: *p16/CDKN2* and *p14*^{ARF} (discussed below).

The most frequently overrepresented chromosome arm is 5p [21], which encodes SKP2 (5p13), a protein involved in control of the cell cycle.

Tumor Suppressor Gene Inactivation in Mesothelioma

Tumor suppressor gene protein products are involved in the negative control of cell proliferation and in positive control of apoptosis. Tumor suppressor gene expression in tumors is altered by inactivating point mutations, aberrant expressions, epigenetic silencing most often caused by methylation of their 5′ end and gene rearrangements, monoallelic or complete gene loss (homozygous deletion), and combinations of these factors. All of the cytogenetic abnormalities and deletion sites are likely to be involved in inactivation of tumor suppressor genes in mesothelial tumorigenesis. However, current knowledge confirms a pathogenetic role only for the following tumor suppressor genes in malignant mesothelioma: CDK-inhibitors *p16*^{INK4A}, *p53*, and *NF2*.

P16^{INK4}, an encoded protein at the smallest region of overlap of 9p21 deletion, is an inhibitor of the cyclin-dependent kinases 4 and 6, and inhibits the catalytic activity of these kinases, which drive Rb phosphorylation. Thus, P16^{INK4} allows Rb to be maintained in an underphosphorylated state, permitting G_1 arrest in binding the transcription factor E2F. Inactivation of P16 in tumors rivals inactivation of P53 as a significant step in carcinogenesis. The most frequent modes of inactivation of P16 are homozygous deletion and methylation, whereas P16 missense mutations are rare. Due to the high frequency of 9p21 homozygous deletion in mesothelioma cell lines, p16^{INK4} has been proposed as a putative tumor suppressor gene in malignant mesothelioma. Although *p16*^{INK4} gene is homozygously deleted in 85% of cell lines, it was homozygously deleted in only 22% of tumor specimens [31, 32]. The *p16* mutations were identified in 2 of 39 mesothelioma cell lines but in no primary tumors. Although genetically normal cells may hinder the ability to detect homozygous deletion, it has been demonstrated that transcriptional repression and silencing of tumor suppressor genes by hypermethylation of their promoter is frequent in various cancers including lung cancer [33]. In one series, *p16* was inactivated, with loss of protein expression demonstrated by immunohistochemistry, in most cases of malignant mesothelioma (tumor and cell lines) [34]. This allows the conclusion that homozygous deletion and methylation of p16, occurs in malignant mesothelioma in vivo and in vitro.

The *p16*^{INK4} 9p21 locus is also the location of another tumor suppressor gene *p14*^{ARF}, the transcription of which starts from a different exon 1β (alternative reading frame, or ARF) and shares with *p16*^{INK4} exons 2 and 3. Both genes induce G_1 arrest when transfected. P14^{ARF} is an essential upstream element for P53 activation in response to aberrant oncogene activation (ras, E2F1, loss of Rb, myc), whereas P16^{INK4} acts on the Rb pathway.

Homozygous loss of both P16 and $P14^{ARF}$ would collectively affect both Rb- and P53-dependent growth regulatory pathways and especially evasion of G_1 arrest. Activation of P53 secondary to DNA damage (induced by asbestos fibers) requires $P14^{ARF}$, suggesting that both $P16^{INK4}$ and $P14^{ARF}$ are the critical targets of 9p21 deletion. $P16^{INK4}$ inactivation correlates with retention of Rb tumor suppressor gene activity in mesothelioma [34–36], as seen in human lung tumors [37, 38].

p53 *Alterations in Malignant Mesothelioma*

The *p53* gene maps at chromosome 17p13 [39], where loss of heterozygosity is rare in human mesotheliomas, in contrast with the high frequency of rearrangement (76%) in murine mesothelioma [40]. Despite a low incidence of LOH at the *p53* 17p13 location, P53 stabilization detected by immunohistochemistry, reflecting *p53* dysfunction, was found in 25% to 70% of malignant mesotheliomas [41–43]. Because P53 stabilization and immunodetection often reflect *p53* missense mutations, an active search for *p53* mutations in malignant mesothelioma was performed; mutations were rarely found, even in cases of P53 overexpression [44, 45] or in experimental animal models of mesothelioma [46]. Overexpression of P53 in malignant mesothelioma in the absence of mutation suggested the existence of a protein partner that may associate with P53 to stabilize it. MDM2 was evoked because overexpression of MDM2 has been found in one-third of malignant mesotheliomas [43, 47]. Recent results indicate that an increased level of MDM2, a 90-kDa protein, binds P53 and reduces its half-time for inducing proteasome-mediated ubiquitination of P53. This probably explains why there was no relation in various studies between overexpression of MDM2 and the level of stabilization or overexpression of P53 protein. MDM2 overexpression occurred in about one-third of mesothelioma cell lines compared to that in normal human bronchial epithelial cells and normal fibroblasts. This indicates that in these cases overexpression of MDM2 inactivates P53 tumor suppressor activity. MDM2 interferes not only with P53 tumor suppressor activity, but when binding E2F1 it inactivates Rb-dependent G_1 arrest [48, 49]. Exposure of normal human mesothelial cells or mesothelial lines expressing wild-type P53 to ionizing radiation induced nuclear accumulation of P53 and its target gene $p21^{waf1}$, indicating that the P53 protein detected by immunohistochemical staining was responsive to DNA damage and was transcriptionally active at least partly in most mesothelial cells. The variation observed in *MDM2* gene expression was not considered biologically significant overexpression, being at most five times more than that of normal cells. In conclusion, MDM2 protein is probably not a major factor in the etiology of malignant mesothelioma. Another means of P53 inactivation could be the occurrence of the expression of SV40 large Tag, as SV40-infected cells expressed high levels of wild-type P53 protein.

Simian Virus 40, a Large T Antigen in Human Mesothelioma: Its Role in Tumor Suppressor Gene Activation

Studies of DNA tumor viruses, such as simian virus 40 (SV40), have shown that virally encoded large T antigen (Tag) of SV40 promotes transformation of cultured human and rodent cells and induces tumors when expressed as a transgene in mice. This virus causes mesothelioma when injected into the pleural space of hamsters [50]. The complex of Tag with two important tumor suppressor genes *p53* and *Rb*, and with other members of the Rb pocket (P105, P107, PRb2/P130) disrupts normal cell cycle control and presumably antagonizes P53-induced apoptosis. SV40-like DNA sequences were found initially in 60% of mesotheliomas, along with the demonstration of simian virus large T antigen in most. The matching lung samples did not contain SV40-like sequences [51]. This first study suggested that SV40-like virus may act independently or as a co-carcinogen with asbestos (by the polymerase chain reaction, or PCR).

Recently, PCR has also permitted detection of SV40-like DNA sequences in other human tumors including osteosarcomas, ependymomas, and gliomas, raising the possibility that SV40 or related viruses are involved in their etiology. Some studies have provided conflicting information about the role of SV40-like sequences in malignant mesothelioma [44, 52, 53], and one series reported no SV40 Tag in 17 mesothelioma samples [54]. In summary, investigations for SV40-like DNA sequences and immunohistochemistry for small or large Tag have shown 52% to 90% of patients with a mesothelioma from the United States, Italy, and Germany to be SV40-positive [55]. Investigators from the United Kingdom provided evidence for the association of SV40 with human mesothelioma in the British population and postulated that SV40 could have contaminated polio vaccines given between 1959 and 1961, stressing the need for research on SV40 DNA in mesotheliomas diagnosed before this date [56]. Confirmation is awaited.

It has been postulated that SV40 might bind and inactivate wild-type P53 in mesothelioma [57], interfering with DNA repair, apoptotic, and growth inhibitory functions and might in this way contribute to the development of mesothelioma. Another result came from a French study [52] that confirmed the presence of SV40-like DNA sequences by PCR in 47.6% of mesotheliomas and in 16% of nonneoplastic pleural and pulmonary diseases. This raises the possibility that SV40-like sequences may not be related to mesothelioma. In addition, immunohistochemistry using anti-Tag antigen did not demonstrate nuclear staining.

Finally, multiinstitutional studies recently reported the results of DNA protein analysis, SV40 sequences, and SV40 large T antigen expression in 83% of a small number of mesotheliomas (12 cases), and the presence in some patients of both SV40 and asbestos. The authors concluded that these two carcinogens might interact in mesothelioma oncogenesis [58]. The ability of adenovirus vectors expressing antisense to SV40 to induce growth arrest and apoptosis in T antigen-positive human pleural mesothelioma cells was reported in SV40-transformed, T antigen-positive mesothelial cell lines deficient for $P16^{INK4}$ as well as $P14^{ARF}$ expression (COS-7 cells) [59]. Loss of T/t antigen expression was coincident with p21 up-regulation, suggesting that antisense to SV40 allowed restoration of P53-mediated pathways and P53-dependent apoptosis. The suggestion that SV40 oncoprotein contributes to the development of pleural mesothelioma offers a basis for interventions to abrogate their expression with the aim of inducing malignant mesothelioma cell apoptosis. Human mesothelioma cells seem to be unusually susceptible to SV40-mediated transformation and asbestos complemented their transformation [60]. The debate on SV40 relevance in mesothelioma carcinogenesis is not resolved. Although it has been demonstrated that SV40 large T antigen interferes with normal expression of the two "in vitro translated" tumor suppressor genes *p53* and *Rb* in human mesothelioma, it has not been proven that SV40 Tag can inactivate *p53* and *Rb* family gene products in vivo.

NF2 *Inactivation*

NF2 tumor suppressor gene (autosomal dominant gene) resides on chromosome 22, which is frequently altered in mesotheliomas. *NF2* gene encodes a 595-amino-acid protein called schwannomin or merlin (moesin-ezrin-radixin-like protein), a highly conserved family of proteins that connect the cytoskeleton to the plasma membrane. Mutations of *NF2* gene were detected in multiple tumor types related to neurofibromatosis (NF2 disorder) but also in *NF2*-unrelated tumors such as melanoma and breast carcinoma. Merlin inactivation is involved in one-half of sporadic vestibular schwannomas and meningiomas and in malignant mesotheliomas. Lung cancer, particularly small-cell lung carcinoma, showed a high frequency of loss of chromosome 22, *NF2* mutations were specifically found in mesotheliomas (41%) but not in lung cancers [61]. All mutations resulted in a carboxy-terminal truncated and presumably inactive protein (in-frame deletions or premature stop codon). This is consistent with previous evidence that all mutations observed in sporadic cancers, melanomas, breast cancers, meningiomas, and schwannomas were of this type. The absence of merlin in some meningiomas and schwannomas occurs without gene mutation but is caused by abnormal ubiquitination of the protein at the post-transcriptional level. The fact that 22q allele loss is not followed by mutation in resting alleles in lung cancers does not exclude the role of merlin in carcinogenesis.

The predominance of the *NF2* mutation in cases with NF2 allelic loss confirms the classic Knudson "two-hit" model of tumor suppressor gene inactivation in the pathogenesis of malignant mesothelioma. Studies [62, 63] have confirmed the frequent mutation of *NF2* in malignant mesothelioma cell lines. mRNA alterations, not confirmed at the DNA level, suggesting aberrant splicing may constitute an additional mechanism for NF2 inactivation in malignant mesothelioma. When Western blot analysis was performed to reveal nf2 protein using polyclonal antibody specific for the C-terminal region, all the cases exhibiting alteration in the *NF2* genes had no detectable nf2 protein in contrast to 11 malignant mesothelioma cell lines without the *NF2* mutation, where nf2 protein was readily detectable. Seventy-two percent of the cases with loss of *NF2* expression were found to have a 22q12 allelic loss, suggesting that inactivation of the *NF2* gene in malignant mesosthelioma occurs via the "two-hit" classic Knudson mechanism. When several cell lines were examined [63], it was found that the *NF2* gene silencing was restricted to a subset of mesothelioma cell lines. This *NF2* mutation is now considered a progression rather than an initiating event in mesotheliomas. There is no clear evidence at the moment for the function of NF2 in normal cells and the role and timing of its alteration in oncogenesis, as cell lines were studied more often than primary tumors. Tikoo et al. [64] reported that transfection of NF2 suppressed the malignant phenotype of v-Ha-ras-transformed NIH/3T3 cells, suggesting that an antitumor function of *NF2* is involved in the *ras* signal transduction pathway. Although *ras* mutation does not occur in malignant mesotheliomas [46], genetic inhibition might be a means for *ras* pathway alteration. The overall frequency of *NF2* monoallelic loss is significantly more frequent than *NF2* mutation, giving support for a second supressor gene in the 20q chromosomal region that may contribute to the development of a subset of mesotheliomas lacking *NF2* alterations.

Wilms' Tumor-1 Susceptibility Gene

Wilms' tumor gene (*WT1*) encodes a transcription factor with four DNA-binding zinc fingers at the C-terminus and a transactivation domain at the N-terminus. In transfection assays, WT1 represses transcription from promoters of several early growth response genes including IGF-1 receptor (IGF-1R), and EGF receptor (EGF-R) [65]. *WT1*-dependent transcriptional regulation depends on wild-type *p53*, in the absence of which *WT1* could act as a potential repressor of growth factor receptor genes. A link between *WT1* and *p53* and the level of expression of these growth factor genes has been sought in malignant mesotheliomas [66]. However, although *WT1* is expressed in almost all mesotheliomas, in most reactive mesothelial cells and early mesotheliomas with extensive pleural surface growth there was no correlation between WT1 immunostaining and EGF receptors or IGF-1 receptor, and no significant molecular correlation with *p53* expression status in these mesothelial proliferations [67]. *WT1* has not been found to be mutant, except in one exceptional case. It is regarded as the signature of a differentiation state because it is more commonly expressed in epithelial than sarcomatous mesothelioma. *WT1*, which is normally expressed during the development of mesodermal tissues, could be specifically expressed in those tissues undergoing mesenchymal–epithelial transition [68]. At the present, *WT1* cannot be considered a tumor suppressor gene in mesothelioma cells.

Conclusions

Mesothelioma is most often an asbestos-induced disease. Asbestos is responsible for up-regulation of a number of growth factors and cytokine activation as well as chromosomal aberrations in genes regulating the initiation of cell division. The *p53* and *Rb* pathways are almost constantly disrupted in mesotheliomas owing to frequent *p16* inactivation disrupting the *Rb*-dependent G_1 checkpoint. Although *p53* is present in its wild-type state, complexing of P53 with SV40 Tag or with MDM2 is likely to inactivate *p53* at the protein level, reducing the selection pressure for *p53* inactivation at the genetic level. Tag might be required during the initiation of tumor development to mediate *p53* inactivation, which promotes rapid acquisition of further oncogenic genetic alterations. Inactivation of *p53* by Tag or MDM2 in mesothelial cells that suffer asbestos-induced chromosomal damage may allow them to escape *p53*-dependent apoptosis, which may favor oncogenic mutations. However, the ability of Tag and MDM2 to form complexes with "endogenous p53 and pRb protein" and to block cell cycle control and apoptosis in mesothelioma cells in vivo must be demonstrated. *NF2* inactivation is an important stage of mesothelioma oncogenesis probably affecting the *ras* pathway. *WT1* has not been clearly implicated in mesothelioma oncogenesis and is mainly considered a marker of mesothelioma cell differentiation.

References

1. Churg A. Asbestos lung burden and disease patterns in man. In: Gutherie G, Mossman BT (eds) Health effects of mineral dusts: reviews in mineralogy, vol 28. Washington, DC: Mineralogical Society of America; 1993:410–26.
2. Barrettt JC. Cellular and molecular mechanisms of asbestos carcinogenicity: implications for bio-persistence. Environ Health Perspect 1994;102:19–23.
3. Hesterberg TW, Chase G, Axten C, et al. Biopersistence of synthetic vitreous fibers and amosite asbestos in the rat lung following inhalation. Toxicol Appl Pharmacol 1998;151:262–75.
4. Selikoff IJ, Hammond EC, Seidman H. Latency of asbestos disease among insulation workers in the United States and Canada. Cancer 1980;46:2736–40.
5. Hesterberg TW, Barrett JC. Induction by asbestos fibers of anaphase abnormalities: mechanism for aneuploidy induction and possibly carcinogenesis. Carcinogenesis 1985;6:473–5.
6. Olofsson K, Mark J. Specificity of asbestos-induced chromosomal aberrations in short-term cultured human mesothelial cells. Cancer Genet Cytogenet 1989; 41:33–9.

7. Kamp DW, Graceffa P, Prior WA, et al. The role of free radicals in asbestos induced diseases. Free Radic Biol Med 1992;12:293–315.
8. Hardy JA, Aust AE. Iron in asbestos chemistry and carcinogenicity. Chem Rev 1995;95:97–118.
9. Jaurand MC. Mechanims of fiber-induced genotoxicity. Environ Health Perspect 1997;105:1073–84.
10. Soini Y, Kinnula V, Kaarteenaho-Wiik R, et al. Apoptosis and expression of apoptosis regulation proteins bcl-2, mcl-1, bcl-X, and bax in malignant mesothelioma. Clin Cancer Res 1999;5:3508–15
11. Kahlos K, Soini Y, Paakko P, et al. Proliferation, apotosis, and manganese superoxide dismutase in malignant mesothelioma. Int J Cancer 2000;88:37–43.
12. Lauber B, Leuthold M, Schmitter D, et al. An autocrine mitogenic activity produced by a pleural human mesothelioma cell line. Int J Cancer 1992;50: 943–50.
13. Gerwin BI, Lechner JF, Reddel RR, et al. Comparison of properties of transforming growth factor beta and platelet-derived growth factor by normal human mesothelial cells and mesothelioma cell lines. Cancer Res 1987;47:6180–4.
14. Versnel MA, Hagemeijer A, Bouts MJ, et al. Expression of c-sis (PDGF B-chain) and PDGF A-chain genes in ten human malignant mesothelioma cell lines derived from primary and metastatic tumors. Oncogene 1988;2:601–5.
15. Lechner JF, Tesfaigzi J, Gerwin BI. Oncogenes and tumor suppressor genes in mesothelioma-A synopsis. Environ Health Perspect 1997;105:1061–7.
16. Gerwin BI. Cytokine signaling in mesothelial cells: receptor expression closes the autocrine loop. Am J Respir Cell Mol Biol 1996;14:505–7.
17. Tiainen M, Tammilehto L, Mattson K, et al. Non-random chromosomal abnormalities in malignant pleural mesothelioma. Cancer Genet Cytogenet 1988; 33:251–74.
18. Hagemeijer A, Versnel MA, Van Drunnen E, et al. Cytogenetic analysis of malignant mesothelioma. Cancer Genet Cytogenet 1990;47:1–28.
19. Taguchi T, Jhanwar SC, Siegried JM, et al. Recurrent deletions of specific chromosomal sites in 1p, 3p, 6q, and 9p in human malignant mesothelioma. Cancer Res 1993;53:4349–55.
20. Murthy SS, Testa JR. Asbestos, chromosomal deletions, and tumor suppressor gene alterations in human malignant mesothelioma. J Cell Physiol 1999;180: 150–7.
21. Balsara BR, Bell DW, Sonoda G, et al. Comparative genomic hybridization and loss of heterozygosity analyses identify a common region of deletion at 15q11.1–15 in human malignant mesothelioma. Cancer Res 1999;59:450–4.
22. Tiainen M, Tammilehto L, Rautonen J, et al. Chromosomal abnormalities and their correlations with asbestos exposure and survival in patients with mesothelioma. Br J Cancer 1989;60:618–26.
23. Lee WC, Balsara B, Liu Z, et al. Loss of heterozygosity analysis defines a critical region in chromosome 1p22 commonly deleted in human malignant mesothelioma. Cancer Res 1996;56:4297–301.
24. Shivapurkar N, Virmani AK, Wistuba II, et al. Deletions of chromosome 4 at multiple sites are frequent in malignant mesothelioma and small cell lung carcinoma. Clin Cancer Res 1999;5:17–23.
25. Bell DW, Jhanwar SC, Testa JR. Multiple regions of allelic loss from chromosome arm 6q in malignant mesothelioma. Cancer Res 1997;57:4057–62.

26. Theile M, Seitz S, Arnold W, et al. A defined chromosome 6 fragment (at D6S310) harbors a putative tumor suppressor gene for breast cancer. Oncogene 1996;13:677–85.
27. Sandhu AK, Kaur GP, Reddy DE, et al. A gene on 6q14–21 rstores senescence to immortal ovarian tumor cells. Oncogene 1996;12:247–52.
28. Negrini M, Sabbioni S, Possati L, et al. Suppression of tumorigenicity of breast cancer cells by microcell-mediated chromosome transfer: studies on chromosomes 6 and 11. Cancer Res 1994;54:1331–6.
29. Lim D, Hasty P. A mutation in mouse rad51 results in early an embryonic lethal that is suppressed by a mutation in p53. Mol Cell Biol 1996;16:7133–43.
30. Sharan SK, Morimatsu M, Albrecht U, et al. Embryonic lethality and radiation hypersensitivity mediated by Rad51 in mice lacking Brca2. Nature 1997; 386:804–10.
31. Cheng JQ, Jhanwar SC, Kline WM, et al. P16 alterations and deletion mapping of 9p21–p22 in malignant mesothelioma. Cancer Res 1994;54:5547–51.
32. Prins JB, Williamson KA, Kamp MMK, et al. The gene for the cyclin-dependent-kinase-4 inhibitor, CDKN2A, is preferentially deleted in malignant mesothelioma. Int J Cancer 1998;75:649–53.
33. Merlo A, Herman JG, Mao L, et al. 5′ CpG island methylation is associated with transcriptionnal silencing of the tumor suppressor p16/CDKN2/MTS1 in human cancers. Nat Med 1995;686–92.
34. Kratzke RA, Otterson GA, Lincoln CE, et al. Immunohistochemical analysis of the $p16^{INK4}$ cyclin-dependent kinase inhibitor in malignant mesothelioma. J Natl Cancer Inst 1995;87:1870–5.
35. Van Der Meeren A, Seddon MB, Kispert J, et al. Lack of expression of the retinoblastoma gene is not frequently involved in the genesis of human mesothelioma. Eur Respir Rev 1993;3:177–9.
36. Remel M, Segers K, Van Marck E. Differential immunohistochemical staining for retinoblastoma protein with antibodies C15 and IF8 in malignant mesothelioma. Pathol Res Pract 1994;190:138–41.
37. Kratzke RA, Greatens TM, Rubins JB, et al. Rb and $p16^{INK4}$ expression in resected non small cell lung tumors. Cancer Res 1996;56:3415–20.
38. Brambilla E, Moro D, Gazzeri S, et al. Alterations of Rb, $P16^{INK4}$, Cyclin D1 expressions in non small cell lung carcinoma and their clinical significance. J Pathol 1999;188:351–60.
39. Cote RJ, Jhanwar SC, Novick S, et al. Genetic alterations of the p53 gene are a feature of malignant mesotheliomas. Cancer Res 1991;51:5410–16.
40. Cora EM, Kane AB. Alterations in tumor suppressor gene, p53, in mouse mesotheliomas induced by crocidolite asbestos. Eur Respir Rev 1993;3:148–50.
41. Ramael M, Lemmens G, Eerdekens C, et al. Immunoreactivity for p53 protein in malignant mesothelioma and non-neoplastic mesothelium. J Pathol 1992; 168:371–5.
42. Kafiri G, Thomas DM, Shepherd NA, et al. p53 expression is common in malignant mesothelioma. Histopathology 1992;21:331–4.
43. Segers K, Backhovens H, Singh SK, et al. Immunoreactivity for p53 and mdm2 and the detection of p53 mutations in human malignant mesothelioma. Virchows Arch 1995;427:431–16.
44. Metcalf RA, Welsh JA, Bennett WP, et al. P53 and Kirsten-ras mutations in human mesothelioma cell lines. Cancer Res 1992;52:2610–15.

45. Mor O, Yaron P, Huszar M, et al. Absence of p53 mutations in malignant mesothelioma. Am J Respir Cell Mol Biol 1997;16:9–13.
46. Ni Z, Liu Y, Keshava N, et al. Analysis of K-ras and p53 mutations in mesotheliomas from humans and rats exposed to asbestos. Mutat Res 2000;468: 87–92.
47. Ungar S, Van De Meeren A, Tammilehto L, et al. High levels of MDM2 are not correlated with the presence of wild-type p53 in human malignant mesothelioma cell lines. Br J Cancer 1996;74:1534–40.
48. Xiao ZX, Chen J, Levine AJ, et al. Interaction between the retinoblastoma protein and the oncoprotein MDM2. Nature 1995;375:694–8.
49. Martin K, Trouche D, Hagemeier C, et al. Stimulation of E2F1/DP1 transcriptional activity by MDM2 oncoprotein. Nature 1995;375:691–4.
50. Cicala C, Pompetti F, Carbone M. SV40 induces mesotheliomas in hamsters. Am J Pathol 1993;142:1524–34.
51. Carbone M, Pass HI, Rizzo P, et al. Simian virus 40-like DNA sequences in human pleural mesothelioma. Oncogene 1994;9:1781–90.
52. Galateau-Salle F, Bidet P, Iwatsubo Y, et al. SV40-like DNA sequences in pleural mesothelioma, bronchopulmonary carcinoma, and non-malignant pulmonary diseases. J Pathol 1998;184:252–7.
53. De Luca A, Baldi A, Esposito V, et al. The retinoblastoma gene family pRb/p105, p107, pRb2/p130 and simian virus-40 T-antigen in human mesotheliomas. Nat Med 1997;3:913–16.
54. Mulatero C, Surentheran T, Breuer J, et al. Simian virus 40 and human pleural mesothelioma. Thorax 1999;54:60–1.
55. Jasani B, Cristaudo A, Emri SA, et al. Association of SV40 with human tumours. Semin Cancer Biol 2001;11:49–62.
56. Pepper C, Jasani B, Navabi H, et al. Simian virus 40 large T antigen (SV40LTAg) primer specific DNA amplification in human pleural mesothelioma tissue. Thorax 1996;51:1074–6.
57. Carbone M, Rizzo P, Grimley PM, et al. Simian virus-40 large-T antigen binds p53 in human mesotheliomas. Nat Med 1997;3:908–12.
58. Testa JR, Carbone M, Hirvonen A, et al. A multi-institutional study confirms the presence and expression of simian virus 40 in human malignant mesothelioma. Cancer Res 1998;58:4505–9.
59. Waheed I, Guo ZS, Chen GA, et al. Antisense to SV40 early gene region induces growth arrest and apoptosis in T-antigen-positive human pleural mesothelioma cells. Cancer Res. 1999;59:6068–73.
60. Bocchetta M, Di Resta I, Powers A, et al. Human mesothelial cells are unusually susceptible to simian virus 40-mediated transformation and asbestos cocarcinogenicity. Proc Natl Acad Sci USA 2000;97:10214–9.
61. Sekido Y, Pass HI, Bader S, et al. Neurofibromatosis type 2 (NF2) gene is somatically mutated in mesothelioma but not in lung cancer. Cancer Res 1995;55: 1227–31.
62. Cheng JQ, Lee WC, Klein MA, et al. Frequent mutations of NF2 and allelic loss from chromosome band 22q12 in malignant mesothelioma: evidence for a two-hit mechanism of NF2 inactivation. Gene Chromosome Cancer 1999;24:238–42.
63. Deguen B, Goutebroze L, Giovannini M, et al. Heterogeneity of mesothelioma cell lines as defined by altered genomic structure and expression of the NF2 gene. Int J Cancer 1998;77:554–60.

64. Tikoo A, Varga M, Ramesh V, et al. An anti-ras function of neurofibromatosis type 2 gene product (NF2/merlin). J Biol Chem 1994;269:23387–90.
65. Langerak AW, Williamson KA, Hagemeijer A, et al. Expression of the Wilm's tumor gene WT1 in human malignant mesothelioma cell lines and relationship to platelet–derived growth factor a and insulin-like growth factor 2 expression. Genes Chromosomes Cancer 1995;12:87–96.
66. Kumar–Sing S, Segers K, Rodeck U, et al. WT1 mutation in malignant mesothelioma and WT1 immunoreactivity in relation to p53 and growth factor receptor expression, cell type transformation, and prognosis. J Pathol 1997;181: 67–74.
67. Amin KM, Litzky LA, Smythe WR, et al. Wilm's tumor 1 susceptibility (WT1) gene products are selectively expressed in malignant mesothelioma. Am J Pathol 1995;146:344–56.
68. Kumar–Sing S, Jacobs W, Dhaene K, et al. Syndecan-1 expression in malignant mesothelioma: correlation with cell differentitation, WT1 expression and clinical outcome. J Pathol 1998;186:300–5.

3
Serosal Anatomy and Anatomic Distribution of Mesothelioma

The celomic cavity develops early during embryogenesis and is divided by various partitioning membranes into the pleural, pericardial, and peritoneal cavities. The body cavities, lined by tissue referred to as serosa, have a visceral and a parietal layer. The serosal tissue is composed of a layer of epithelioid mesothelial cells, which in the resting state are usually relatively thin, though are occasionally elongated and appear like squamous epithelial cells (Figure 3.1A). Ultrastructurally, they show characteristic long, slender microvilli (Figure 3.2). They are separated by a basal lamina from the underlying stromal tissue (Figure 3.1B), which is composed of elastic fibers, collagen, and deeper spindle cells that have been referred to as multipotential subserosal cells. Mesotheliomas develop from cells forming the serosal tissue [1, 2].

In the normal resting state, the serosal membranes are thin and almost transparent. The visceral pleura measures approximately 0.1 to 0.3 μm thick. The parietal pleura is separated from the chest wall skeletal muscle by fibrofatty tissue (Figure 3.3) and is approximately 0.2 to 0.4 mm thick.

Serosal tissue is one of the most reactive tissues in the body. With the least degree of injury or irritation, epithelioid mesothelial cells, which in the resting state are often squamoid in appearance, become cuboidal, increase in number, and exhibit enlarged nuclei. As discussed below, reactive mesothelial proliferation can be extremely difficult to differentiate from reactive neoplastic mesothelial cells [3, 4]. Multipotential subserosal cells, which may also exhibit reactive proliferation, have histologic, immunohistochemical, and ultrastructural features of myofibroblasts (Figure 3.4). Immunohistochemically, the normal and reactive epithelioid mesothelial cells express keratins 5 through 8 and 14 through 18 [5]. Reactive multipotential subserosal cells characteristically express keratin, actin, and vimentin (Figure 3.5).

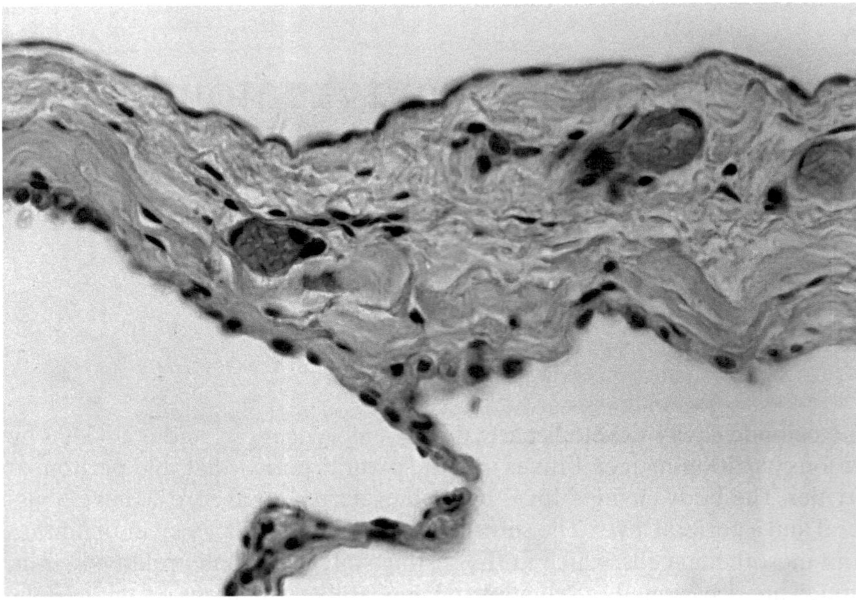

A

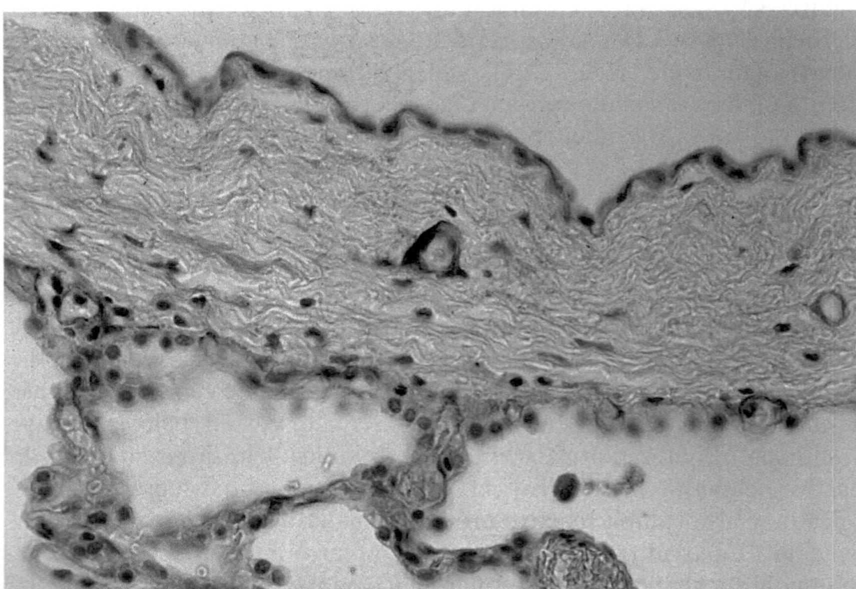

B

FIGURE 3.1. A. Normal visceral pleura is composed of a layer of flattened mesothelial cells and underlying spindle-shaped stromal cells admixed with elastic tissue and collagen. The visceral pleura is approximately 0.1 to 0.3 μm thick. B. Immunohistochemical staining of type IV collagen.

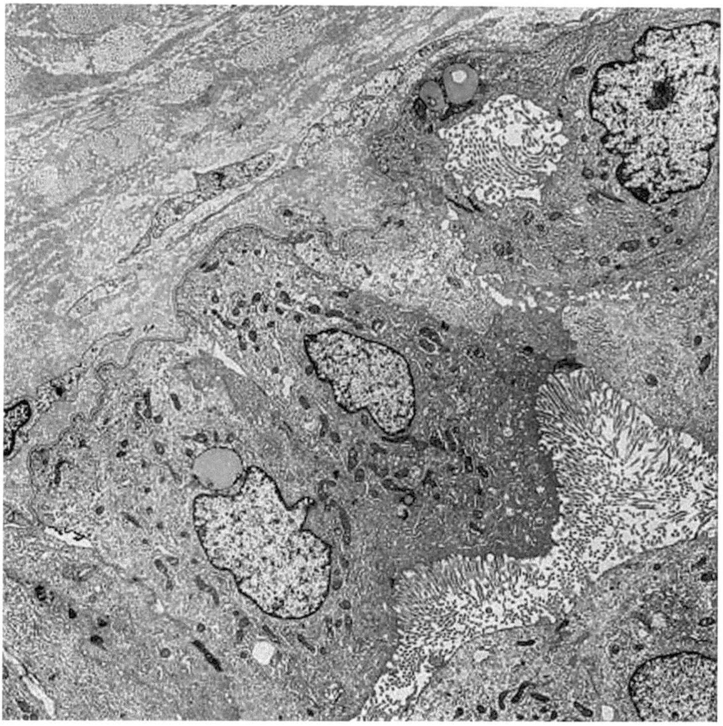

FIGURE 3.2. Ultrastructurally, reactive mesothelial cells typically have long, thin, sinuous microvilli and large nuclei. There are frequent spaces between the adjacent mesothelial cells into which microvilli project.

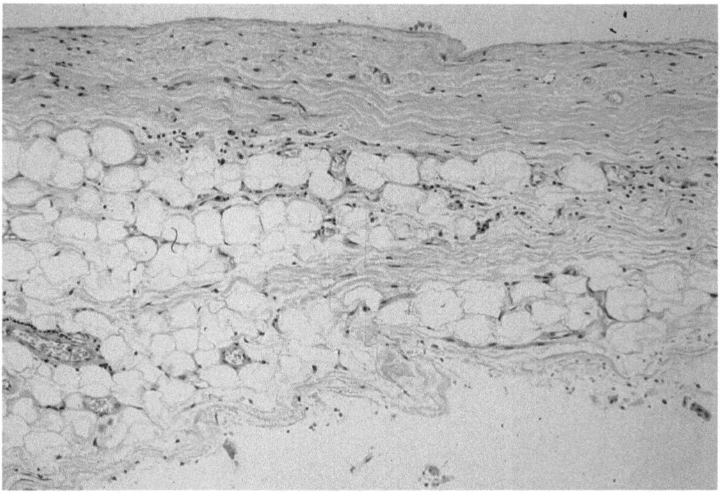

FIGURE 3.3. Parietal pleura is composed of a layer of mesothelial cells and underlying stroma composed of spindle cells, collagen, and elastic tissue. Fibrofatty tissue separates the parietal pleura from the chest wall skeletal muscle. The parietal pleura is approximately 0.2 to 0.4 μm thick.

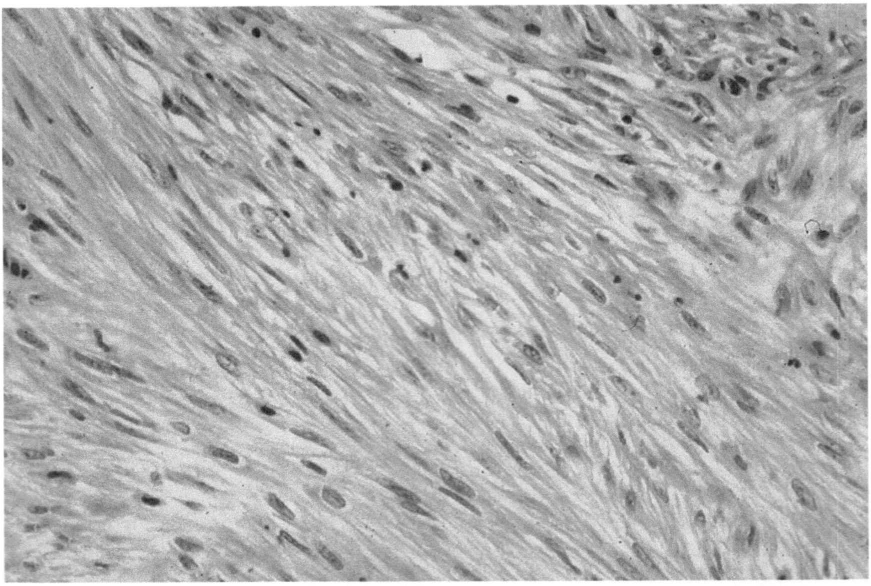

FIGURE 3.4. Spindle stromal cells of serosal membranes lining body cavities are extremely reactive.

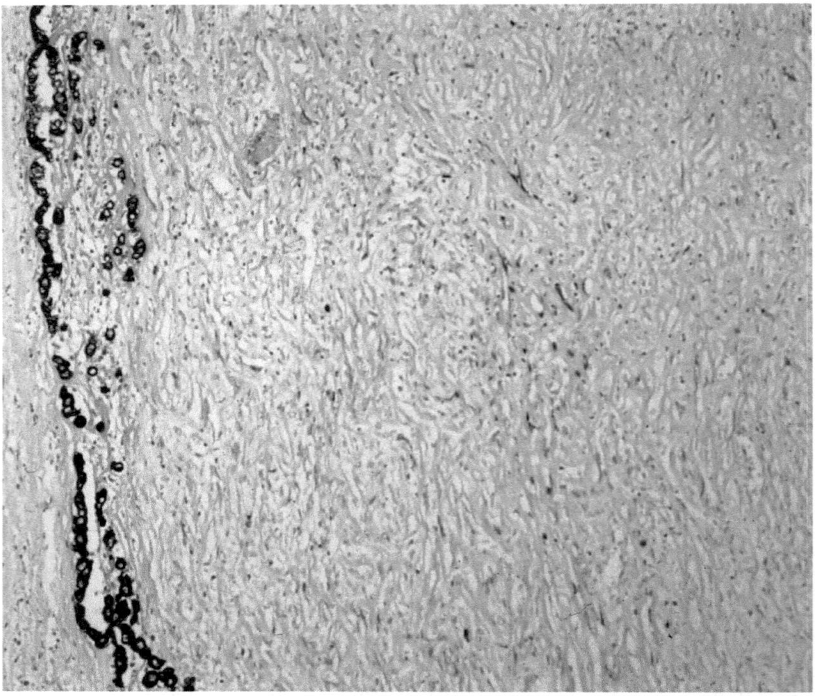

FIGURE 3.5. Reactive serosal membrane stromal cells are expressing cytokeratin underneath a layer of reactive mesothelial cells, which show strong cytokeratin staining. Ultrastructurally, reactive serosal membrane stromal cells have the features of myofibroblasts.

Anatomic Distribution of Mesothelioma

From the Mesopath registry of data for men, more than 90% of mesotheliomas affect the pleural cavities, 6% are peritoneal, and less than 1% affect the pericardium or the tunica vaginalis testis. These figures may be different in other registries. The greater frequency of pleural mesotheliomas in comparison to those in the peritoneum appears to correlate with gender differences regarding the frequency of occupational exposure to asbestos: A smaller proportion of mesotheliomas arise in the pleura in women; and in fact, in one study of Swedish insulation workers, all seven mesotheliomas arose in the peritoneum. Apart from a few cohorts, primary asbestos-induced mesothelioma affects the pleura more often than the peritoneum, in a ratio from 3:1 to 11:1 or more. For men in Australia, 94% of these lesions are pleural mesotheliomas versus 5% located in the peritoneal cavity; for women, the corresponding figures are about 86% and 14%, respectively [6]. The same high ratio of pleural to peritoneal tumors is encountered in the United States [7]. This ratio also varies with industry. In general, the proportion of peritoneal mesotheliomas increases as exposure to commercial amphiboles increases, so the highest proportion of mesotheliomas have been reported in laggers and asbestos manufacturing workers [8, 9]. The incidence of asbestosis is higher among those with peritoneal lesions than in those with pleural tumors [9].

One might expect mesotheliomas unrelated to asbestos to occur with about equal frequency in the pleura and peritoneum. Possible explanations for the higher proportion of peritoneal mesotheliomas in some series and in women include the following: (1) the high proportion of pleural mesotheliomas in men is attributable to past occupational exposure to asbestos, with deposition and translocation of asbestos fibers to a site in anatomic proximity, so asbestos appears to skew the proportional distribution of mesothelioma toward the pleura compared to other sites that involve a more circuitous route for translocation of fibers; (2) a high proportion of peritoneal tumors in some series may be a consequence of patterns of referral for cases that constitute problems in diagnosis because the diagnosis of peritoneal mesothelioma is, in general, more difficult than for pleural mesotheliomas; (3) there may be genuine biologic differences in the inhaled dose, deposition, or transport of different asbestos fiber types in some groups of workers; (4) the exposure response relations for mesothelioma and asbestosis are nonlinear, with the risk of pleural mesothelioma increasing relatively more steeply at low exposures but less steeply at high exposures; thus when an occupation results in relatively low exposure the risk of pleural mesothelioma is increased but without any effect on peritoneal mesothelioma, whereas at high exposure the risk of both increases, but peritoneal mesotheliomas increase disproportionately [9]. The latter would explain the higher asbestos lung fiber burdens observed in the lungs of patients with peritoneal lesions compared to those with pleural lesions [10].

References

1. Whitaker D, Manning LS, Robinson BWS, et al. The pathology of the mesothelium. In: Henderson DW, Shilkin KB, Langlois SLP, et al (eds) Malignant mesothelioma. New York: Hemisphere; 1991;25–68.
2. Bolen JW, Hammar SP, McNutt MA. Reactive and neoplastic serosal tissue: a light microscopic, ultrastructural and immunohistochemical study. Am J Surg Pathol 1986;10:34–47.
3. Henderson DW, Shilkin KB, Whitaker D. Reactive mesothelial hyperplasia versus mesothelioma, including mesothelioma in situ. Am J Clin Pathol 1998; 110:397–404.
4. Churg A, Colby TV, Cagle P, et al. The separation of benign and malignant mesothelial cell proliferations. Am J Surg Pathol 2000;24:1183–2000.
5. Moll R. Cytokeratins as markers of differentiation in the diagnosis of epithelial tumors. Subcell Biochem 1998;31:205–62.
6. Leigh J, Davidson P, Hendrie L, et al. Malignant mesothelioma in Australia 1945–2000. J Occup Health Safety Aust NZ 2001;17:453–70.
7. McDonald AD. Epidemiology of mesothelioma from estimated incidence. Prev Med 1997;6:426–46.
8. Browne K, Smither WJ. Asbestos-related mesothelioma: factors discriminating between pleural and peritoneal sites. Br J Ind Med 1983;40:145–52.
9. Coggon D, Inskip H, Winter P, et al. Differences in occupational mortality from pleural cancer, peritoneal cancer and asbestosis. Occup Environ Med 1995; 52:775–7.
10. Roggli VL, Oury TD, Sporn TA (eds). Pathology of asbestos-associated diseases, 2nd edition. New York: Springer-Verlag; 2004.

4
Clinical Aspects of Mesothelioma

The most common presenting symptoms of malignant pleural mesotheliomas (MPMs) are dyspnea and chest wall pain [1]. They may be associated with constitutional symptoms as well, especially weight loss, malaise, and sometimes night sweats. Additional clinical features include chills, sweats, weakness, fatigue, fever, and anorexia [2].

The frequencies of each symptom, which have been derived from a recent study of 219 patients, are summarized in Table 4.1. Spontaneous pneumothorax is an unusual presenting finding of mesothelioma, with only a few patients presenting this way in most studies [2–9]. Among the 219 patients, 23 had mass lesions, segmental or lobar pulmonary collapse radiologically, or both. Two patients with mediastinal invasion had signs consistent with their disease, namely hoarseness (recurrent laryngeal nerve palsy) and facial swelling (superior vena caval obstruction). Less common features were hoarseness, myalgias, aphonia, dysphagia, abdominal distension, nausea, and a bad taste in the mouth [9].

Clinical Behavior

Irrespective of the histologic type, most patients die within 1 year of presentation. Rarely, patients survive up to 3 years [10], and even more rarely survival may exceed 10 years after histologic diagnosis. Young age, low stage, female sex under age 50, and good performance status are favorable prognostic factors [7, 10–23]. Chest pain as a presenting symptom may be associated with a shorter survival [15–17]. Dyspnea at presentation is also a poor prognostic factor [7, 16, 17]. In one study [18] there was a survival advantage for patients with dyspnea alone, without chest pain. Ruffie et al. [7] and Herndon et al. [17] also demonstrated that weight loss was associated with a poorer prognosis. There was a trend toward pain being more frequently associated with the sarcomatoid subtype. The presence of clinically apparent metastatic disease at presentation was also significantly more common in the sarcomatoid subtype.

TABLE 4.1. Summary of less common presenting symptoms in patients subsequently diagnosed as having MPM.

Clinical presentation	No. of patients[a]
Pneumothorax[b]	8 (3.6%)
Metastatic disease	7 (3.2%)
Incidental/radiologic[c]	4 (1.8%)
Empyema[d]	4 (1.8%)
Other respiratory symptoms[e]	3 (1.4%)
Chest wall disease	3 (1.4%)
Mediastinal disease[f]	2 (0.9%)
"Acute abdomen"[g]	2 (0.9%)
Anemia	2 (0.9%)
Diabetic complications	1 (0.5%)
Total	36 (16.4%)

MPM, malignant pleural mesothelioma.
[a] Percent expressed in relation to the total number of patients ($n = 219$).
[b] Another three patients developed pneumothorax during the illness.
[c] Pleural disease was noted on the chest radiograph obtained for unrelated reasons.
[d] Temperature, malaise, and signs of pleural thickening following a chest infection.
[e] Cough ($n = 2$) and hemoptysis ($n = 1$) were seen in the absence of any other respiratory symptoms.
[f] Recurrent laryngeal nerve palsy ($n = 1$) and superior vena caval obstruction ($n = 1$) were present.
[g] Patients presented to general surgeons with abdominal and chest signs.

Table 4.2 lists studies that examined survival in relation to presenting symptoms.

Few studies have investigated the association of prognosis with histologic subtype [7, 10, 15, 17, 19–26]. The epithelioid subtype appears to be associated with a longer survival after diagnosis than the biphasic or sarcomatoid subtype.

Radiology

Frequent presenting radiologic findings include pleural thickening, effusion, and pleural masses. A rare presentation is with miliary pulmonary parenchymal involvement, resembling tuberculosis [11]. Other asbestos-related abnormalities may be present, such as pleural plaques, which were identified in 70% of patients in one series [12], and asbestosis. Rarely, a coexistent primary pulmonary carcinoma may be seen [13]. Pulmonary emphysema is common, as these patients often smoke.

TABLE 4.2. Summary of studies that have evaluated the influence of presenting symptoms on survival of MPM patients.

Study	Year	No. in study	Pain (%)	SOB (%)	Weight loss (%)	Survival analysis[a]
Alberts [20]	1988	262	58	74	2.6	NS
Antman [15]	1988	136	48	60	15	Pain: $p < 0.001$[b]
Calavrezos [16]	1988	132	72	88	—	Pain: $p = 0.003$ SOB: $p = 0.03$
Hulks [18]	1989	68	47	67	23	Pain vs. SOB: $p < 0.01$
Ruffie [7]	1989	332	33[c]	28[c]	—	Pain: NS SOB: $p = 0.001$ Weight: $p = 0.001$
Tammilehto [22]	1992	98[d]	47	46	—	NS
Manzini [24]	1993	80	51	65	23	NS
Fusco [23]	1993	113	55	65	14	NS
Yates [21]	1997	272	38[e] (+)	33[e] (–)	—	NS
Herndon [17]	1998	257[f]	60 ($n = 219$)	70 ($n = 216$)	41 ($n = 212$)	Pain: $p < 0.001$ SOB: $p = 0.03$ Weight: $p = 0.004$
Current study	2003	219	42	55	9	NS

NS, not statistically significant at the 5% level.
[a] Log-rank statistic unless otherwise specified.
[b] Cox regression.
[c] Another 29% of patients had both symptoms.
[d] Includes five peritoneal cases.
[e] Stratification includes the presence (+) or absence (–) of effusion.
[f] Symptoms were not recorded for all cases.

Computed tomography (CT) is more sensitive than plain chest radiographs for detecting pulmonary fibrosis as well as for determining the extent of the pleural abnormalities and involvement of adjacent structures [14] (Figures 4.1 and 4.2).

Laboratory Findings

The pleural aspirate is an exudate, and the glucose and pH may be reduced. The fluid in epithelioid mesotheliomas may be viscid owing to large amounts of hyaluronic acid (Figure 4.3). Hematologic abnormalities include increased erythrocyte sedimentation rate, fibrinogen, and platelets.

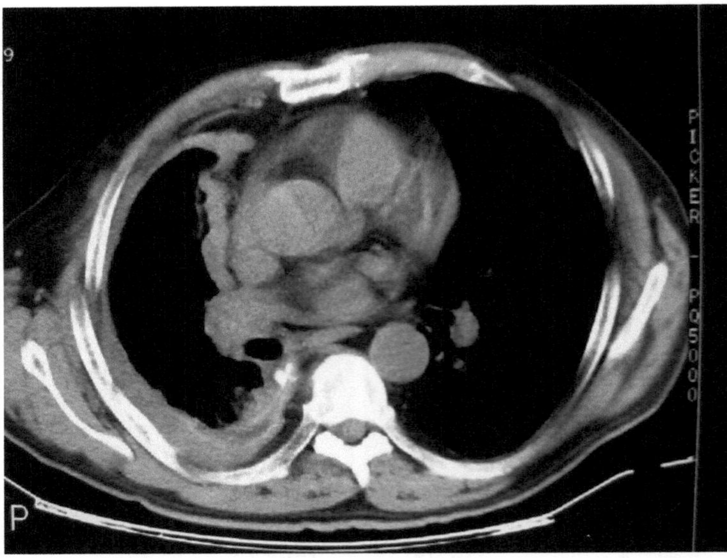

FIGURE 4.1. Computed tomography of the thorax from a patient showing diffuse, irregular thickening of a malignant diffuse mesothelioma with retraction of the hemithorax.

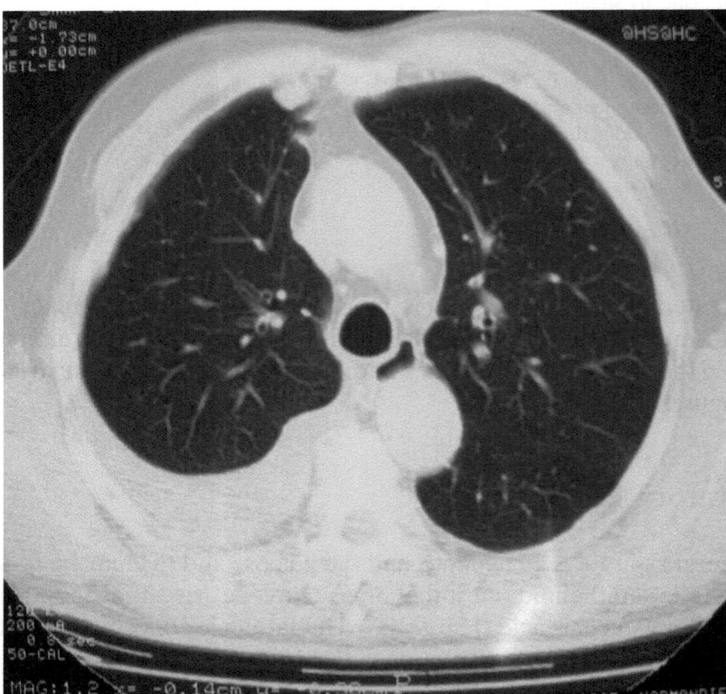

FIGURE 4.2. Computed tomography of the thorax from a patient presenting a diffuse malignant mesothelioma with pleural effusion.

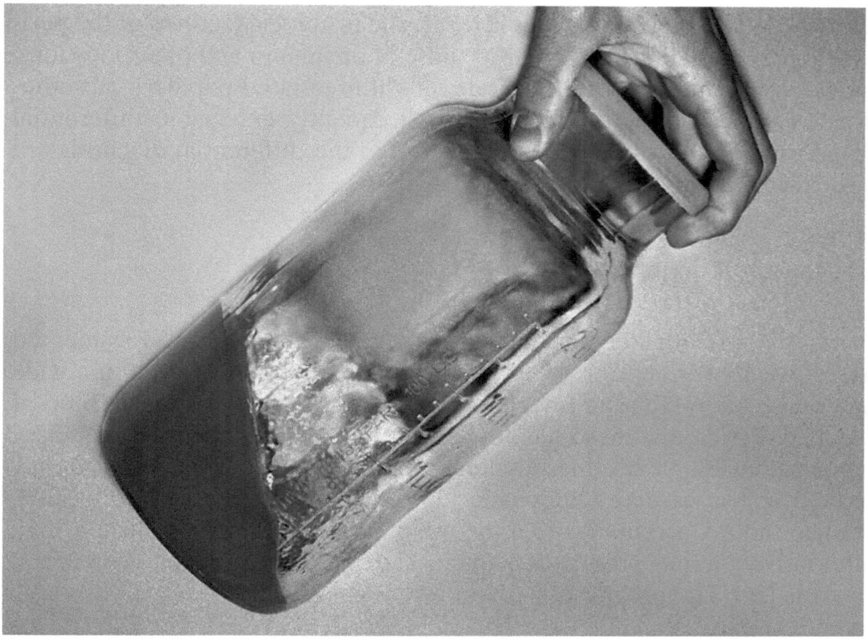

FIGURE 4.3. In epithelioid mesotheliomas the fluid may be viscid owing to large amounts of hyaluronic acid.

Peritoneal Mesothelioma

Peritoneal mesotheliomas are rarer than the pleural variety and 32% of cases are associated with asbestosis [27]; in fact, 85% of these patients give a history of asbestos exposure. Most patients are male, the average age being 44.7 years (range 18 to 49 years) [28]. The presenting symptoms are often vague and consist of abdominal pain and gastrointestinal disturbances, including dysphagia. In one recent report, four cases presented as localized acute inflammatory lesions, acute appendicitis, acute cholecystitis, and an incarcerated umbilical hernia, respectively [29]. The diagnosis was only made on histology. Ascites and palpable masses may develop owing to diffuse peritoneal involvement and weight loss [28]. Invasion of surrounding viscera and metastases were common. Rarely, mesotheliomas present as ovarian masses (see below) [30]. CT is of little value in quantifying the disease [31]. There is doubt as to the wisdom of laparoscopy for diagnosing peritoneal mesothelioma, as the tumor may subsequently grow through the abdominal incisions. Little literature exists on staging in this disease. Survival is 7 months (range 1 to 100 months) for men and 9 months for women (range 0.25 to 49 months) [27, 28]. The epithelioid and myxoid subtypes have more favorable prognoses [27, 28]. The histologic features of the peritoneal mesothelioma are similar to those in the pleura and other locations. However, compared to the pleural well-differentiated papillary mesothelioma, multicystic mesothelioma more frequently enters the differential diagnosis, and the carcinomas considered in the differential diagnosis are also somewhat different (see below).

Pericardial Mesothelioma

Pericardial mesothelioma is rare, and in one review there was documented asbestos exposure in only 14% of cases [32]. The tumor is seen in a wide age range, 12 to 77 years (mean 47 years). There is a male/female ratio of 2:1 [32]. Pericardial mesothelioma must be distinguished from secondary involvement by pleural mesothelioma into the pericardium. Patients may have dyspnea, cardiac tamponade [33, 34], constrictive pericarditis [34], cardiac failure, arrythmias [33], or tumor invading the right atrium [35]; alternatively, it may present as a left atrial thrombus in a patient with mitral stenosis [36]. The prognosis is poor.

Mesothelioma of the Tunica Vaginalis

Mesothelioma of the tunica vaginalis presents as a hydrocele, with or without an associated mass. in one recent series, 1 of 11 patients had a history of asbestos exposure [37]. Follow-up was available for seven patients, who had variable clinical outcomes, with a mean 26-month survival from diagnosis; survival of more than 3 years was recorded for three of the seven, the longest being 15 years. In another series of three patients, one had a history of asbestos exposure and one was alive 3 years after diagnosis [38]. This tumor must be distinguished from secondary spread from a peritoneal mesothelioma [39].

Ovarian Mesothelioma

Primary mesotheliomas of the ovary comprised 0.03% (three cases) of mesothelioma deaths in one UK series [40]. The criteria for the diagnosis of ovarian mesothelioma included the presence of unilateral or bilateral ovarian enlargement, parenchymal replacement in the absence of significant peritoneal disease, or both. Most ovarian mesotheliomas are due to secondary involvement [30, 40]. In approximately 50% of cases, the tumor shows a similar age distribution (with median onset during the sixth decade) and a similar association with asbestos similar to other mesotheliomas. The clinical presentation is usually abdominal or pelvic pain or abdominal swelling, with an adnexal mass found on pelvic examination or at laparotomy. All tumors present as localized masses. Histology is usually epithelioid, with papillary, tubular-glandular, and solid patterns, although a biphasic pattern may be seen. Follow-up in five cases revealed that three patients had died of tumor at postoperative intervals of 8 to 44 months, one was alive with persistent tumor at 18 months, and one was alive with no clinical evidence of tumor at 11 years [30], although in the latter series only two cases were primary ovarian mesotheliomas.

Mesotheliomas should be staged. Various methods of staging have been proposed in the International literature, including the Butchart (IMIG) and Sugerbaker classifications. These classifications may be found among the appendices to this volume. No curative treatment exists at the present time.

References

1. Hasleton PS. Pleural disease. In: Spencer's pathology of the lung, 5th edition. New York: McGraw Hill; 1996.
2. Adams VI, Unni KK, Muhm JR, Jett JR, Ilstrup DM, Bernatz PE. Diffuse malignant mesothelioma of pleura: diagnosis and survival in 92 cases. Cancer 1986;58:1540–51.
3. Law M, Hodson M, Turner-Warick M. Malignant mesothelioma of the pleura: clinical aspects and symptomatic treatment. Eur J Respir Dis 1984;65:162–8.
4. Boutin C, Rey F, Gouvernet J, et al. Thoracoscopy in pleural malignant mesothelioma: a prospective study of 188 consecutive patients. Cancer 1993;72:394–404.
5. Jordan K, Kwong J, Flint J, et al. Surgically treated pneumothorax. Chest 1997; 111:280–5.
6. Mannes G, Gouw A, Berendsen H, et al. Mesothelioma presenting with pneumothorax and interlobar tumour. Eur Respir J 1991;4:120–1.
7. Ruffie P, Feld R, Minkin S, Cormier Y, Boutan-Laroze A, Ginsberg R, et al. Diffuse malignant mesothelioma of the pleura in Ontario and Quebec: a retrospective study of 332 patients. J Clin Oncol 1989;7:1157–68.
8. Sheard J, Taylor W, Soorae A, et al. Pneumothorax and malignant mesothelioma in patients over the age of 40. Thorax 1991;46:584–5.
9. Walz R, Koch H. Malignant pleural mesothelioma: some aspects of epidemiology, differential diagnosis and prognosis. Pathol Res Pract 1990;186:124–34.
10. Mark EJ, Shin DH. Diffuse malignant mesothelioma of the pleura: a clinicopathological study of six patients with a prolonged symptom-free interval or extended survival after biopsy and a review of the literature of long-term survival. Virchows Arch A Pathol Anat Histopathol 1993;422:445–51.
11. Musk A. More cases of miliary mesothelioma. Chest 1995;108:587.
12. Roggli VL, Sharma A, Butnor KJ, et al. Malignant mesothelioma and occupational exposure to asbestos: a clinicopathological correlation of 1445 cases. Ultrastruct Pathol 2002;26:55–65.
13. Attanoos RL, Thomas DH, Gibbs AR. Synchronous diffuse malignant mesothelioma and carcinomas in asbestos-exposed individuals. Histopathology 2003; 43:387–92.

14. Kreel L. Computed tomography in mesothelioma. Semin Oncol 1981;8:302–12.
15. Antman K, Shemin R, Ryan L, et al. Malignant mesothelioma: prognostic variables in a registry of 180 patients, the Dana-Faber Cancer Institute and Brigham and Women's Hospital experience over two decades, 1965–1985. J Clin Oncol 1988;6:147–53.
16. Calavrezos A, Koschel G, Husselmann H, et al. Malignant mesothelioma of the pleura: a prospective therapeutic study of 132 patients from 1981–1985. Klin Wochenschr 1988;66:607–13.
17. Herndon J, Green M, Chahinian A, et al. Factors predictive of survival among 337 patients with mesothelioma treated between 1984 and 1994 by the Cancer and Leukaemia Group B. Chest 1998;113:723–31.
18. Hulks G, Thomas J, Waclawski E. Malignant pleural mesothelioma in western Glasgow 1980–6. Thorax 1989;44:496–500.
19. Rusch VW, Venkatraman ES. Important prognostic factors in patients with malignant pleural mesothelioma, managed surgically. Ann Thorac Surg 1999; 68:1799–804.
20. Alberts A, Falkson G, Goedhals L, et al. Malignant pleural mesothelioma: a disease unaffected by current therapeutic maneuvers. J Clin Oncol 1988;6:527–35.
21. Yates D, Corrin B, Stidolph P, et al. Malignant mesothelioma in south east England: clinicopathological experience of 272 cases. Thorax 1997;52:507–12.
22. Tammilehto L. Malignant mesothelioma: prognostic factors in a prospective study of 98 patients. Lung Cancer 1992;8:175–84.
23. Fusco V, Ardizzoni A, Merlo F, et al. Malignant pleural mesothelioma: multivariate analysis of prognostic factors on 113 patients. Anticancer Res 1993;13:683–90.
24. De Pangher Manzini V, Brollo A, Franceschi S, et al. Prognostic factors of malignant mesothelioma of the pleura. Cancer 1993;72:410–7.
25. Spirtas R, Connelly RR, Tucker MA. Survival patterns for malignant mesothelioma: the SEER experience. Int J Cancer 1988;41:525–30.
26. Neumann V, Rutten A, Scharmach M, et al. Factors influencing long-term survival in mesothelioma patients: results of the German mesothelioma register. Int Arch Occup Environ Health 2004;77:191–9.
27. Attanoos RL, Gibbs AR. Peritoneal mesothelioma: Clinicopathological analysis of 227 cases from the U.K. Mesothelioma Register. Arch Anat Cytol Pathol 1998:376.
28. Van Gelder T, Hoogsteden HC, Versnel MA, et al. Malignant peritoneal mesothelioma: a series of 19 cases. Digestion 1989;43:222–7.
29. Kerrigan SAJ, Cagle P, Churg A. Malignant mesothelioma of the peritoneum presenting as an inflammatory lesion: a report of four cases. Am J Surg Pathol 2003;27:248–53.
30. Clement P, Young R, Scully R. Malignant mesotheliomas presenting as ovarian masses: a report of nine cases, including two primary ovarian mesotheliomas. Am J Surg Pathol 1996;20:1067–80.
31. Guest PJ, Reznek RH, Selleslag D, et al. Peritoneal mesothelioma: the role of computed tomography in diagnosis and follow up. Clin Radiol 1992;45: 79–84.
32. Thomason R, Schlegel W, Lucca M, et al. Primary malignant mesothelioma of the pericardium: case report and literature review. Tex Heart Inst J 1994; 21:170–4.

33. Turk J, Kenda M, Kranjeck I. Cardiac tamponade caused by primary pericardial mesothelioma. N Engl J Med 1991;325:814.
34. Watanabe A, Sakata J, Kawamura H, et al. Primary pericardial mesothelioma presenting as constrictive pericarditis: a case report. Jpn Circ J 2000;64:385–8.
35. Lin TS, Chen MF, Lee YT. Pericardial mesothelioma with intracardiac invasion into the right atrium. Cardiology 1994;85:357–60.
36. Miyamoto Y, Nakano S, Shimazaki Y, et al. Pericardial mesothelioma presenting as left atrial thrombus in a patient with mitral stenosis. Cardiovasc Surg 1996;4:51–2.
37. Jones M, Young R, Scully R. Malignant mesothelioma of the tunica vaginalis: a clinicopathologic analysis of 11 cases with review of the literature. Am J Surg Pathol 1995;19:815–25.
38. Plas E, Riedl CR, Pfluger H. Malignant mesothelioma of the tunica vaginalis testis: review of the literature and assessment of pronostic parameters. Cancer 1998;83:2437–46.
39. King JA, Tucker JA, Wong SW. Mesothelioma: a study of 22 cases. South Med J 1997;90:199–205s.
40. Attanoos RL, Gibbs AR. Primary malignant gonadal mesotheliomas and asbestos. Histopathology 2000;37:150–9.

5
Management of Malignant Serosal Effusions

Finding the etiology of a pleural effusion is an every-day challenge for chest physicians [1]. Whereas tuberculosis remains the leading cause of pleural exudates in the Third World, malignancy comes first in Western countries. Whenever pleurisy is found, a sample of pleural fluid must be obtained for inspection as well as odor, chemical analysis, cultures for bacteria and acid-fast bacilli, and cytology, including a search for tumor cells [2]. Its appearance may suggest malignancy at first sight: whereas a light yellow fluid gives no clue, a hemorrhagic one is more suggestive of underlying cancer; a chylous fluid suggests lymphoma; and although rare, a highly viscous orange fluid is quite typical of diffuse malignant mesothelioma. Biochemistry is not diagnostic of malignancy. Although it characterizes an exudate, sometimes with an elevated hyaluronic acid, it suggests but does not prove the presence of a diffuse malignant mesothelioma [3]. A low protein level of less than 20 g/L rules out an underlying pleural disease. Cytologic examination is essential but strongly linked to the pathologist's experience [4–6]. Blind needle biopsies with an Abram's or a Castelain's needle have a low diagnostic yield for malignancy [7–9] but are excellent for assessing pleural tuberculosis [10–12].

Thoracoscopy

Thoracoscopy [13–20] is not a new technique. Jacobaeus invented it in 1910 in Stockhom [21], and over the next 45 years it was used to ensure a successful outcome of therapeutic pneumothorax in tuberculosis patients (Figure 5.1) [22]. With the discovery of streptomycin in 1945, *p*-aminosalicylic acid in 1949, and isoniazid in 1952, there came a sudden decline in the indications for thoracoscopy [23]. This did not last long because with the invention of new technology, including video control, thoracoscopy came back with a wide range of indications—except tuberculosis [24].

The procedure allows visual inspection of the cavity. In some instances, fibrinous veils or bridges must first be torn using the biopsy forceps to break

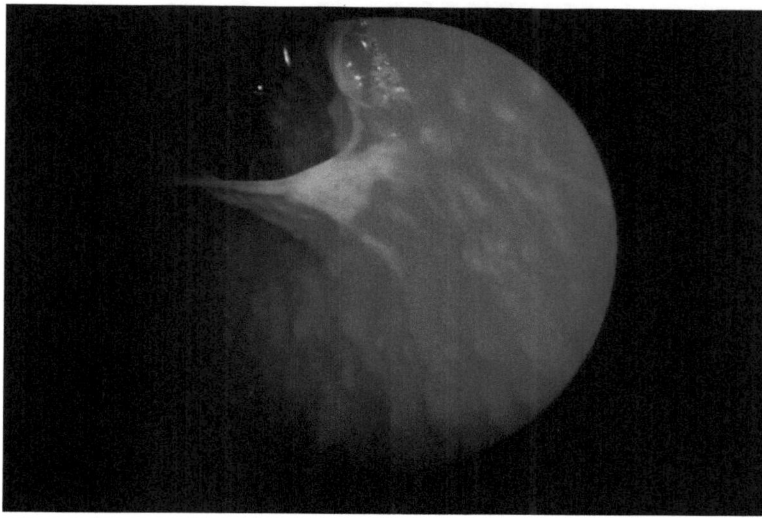

FIGURE 5.1. Tuberculosis showing strands of inflammatory exudates and an adhesion.

through loculated fluid collections but avoiding the ripping off of potentially vascularized adhesions between the lung and the inner chest wall. Such adhesions are more likely to be present when thoracoscopy is delayed: the earlier the procedure is performed, the easier and safer it is with the best diagnostic and therapeutic results.

Minor complications are not exceptional [25]: pain following insufflation of talc; fever that may appear during the following days (usually due to the inflammatory response to talc, but infection must be excluded); subcutaneous emphysema; and local infection at the point of entry (avoided by an appropriate follow-up).

In contrast, major complications are rare. Thoracoscopy is associated with a very low mortality rate, around 1/1000 procedures [26, 27]. Major complications are avoided by strict rules of prevention. Two complications may be difficult to predict: (1) acute respiratory failure may follow insufflation of talc within 36 hours and require steroid therapy; and (2) poor reexpansion of the lung resulting in chronic hydropneumothorax, sometimes associated with persistent air leakage. This complication is more likely to occur in cases of pulmonary atelectasis or carcinomatous lymphangitis.

Asbestos-related benign lesions may have a typical macroscopic appearance, such as the pearly white enamel-like parietal pleural plaques (Figure 5.2); or there may be no specific features such as diffuse pleural thickening. Malignant mesothelioma can be associated with this lesion so that careful examination of the surrounding parietal pleura is necessary in order to detect it (Figure 5.3).

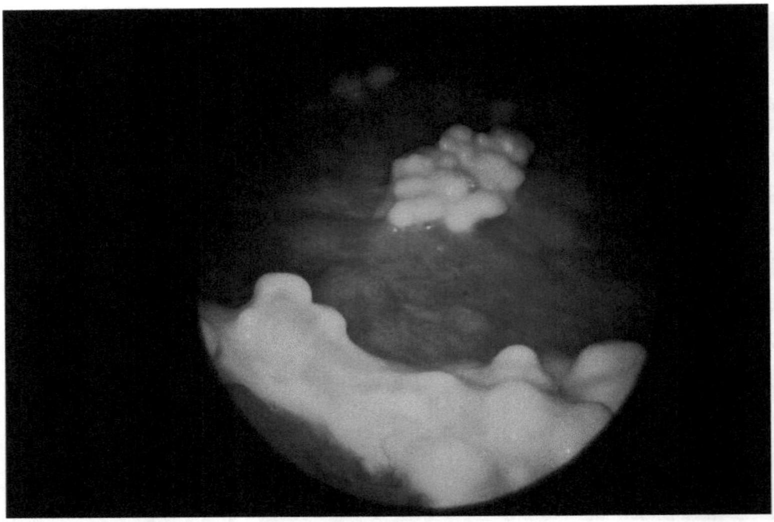

FIGURE 5.2. Thoracoscopic appearance of pearly pleural plaques with adjacent malignant mesothelioma.

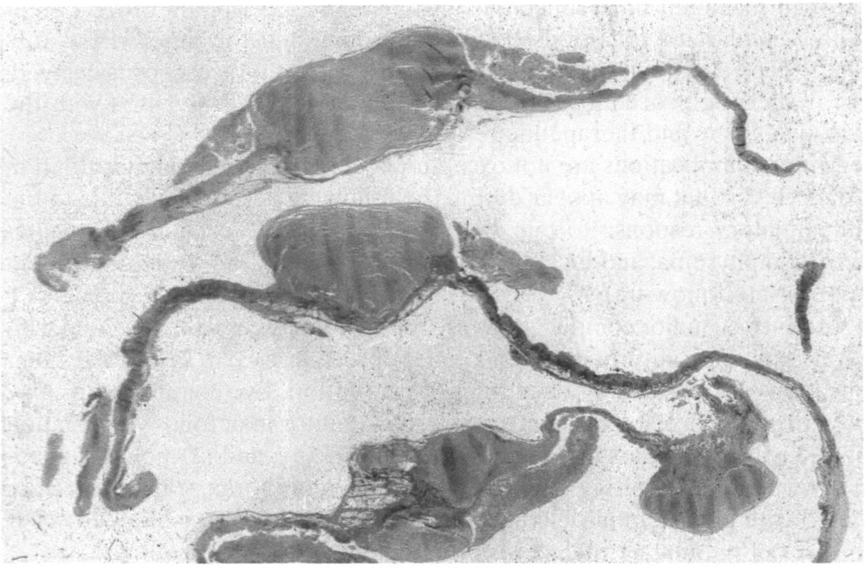

FIGURE 5.3. Thoracoscopic biopsy of the same case showing a superficial epithelioid mesothelioma located at the edge of the pleural plaque.

Thoracoscopy is of great diagnostic value for malignant mesothelioma because it can provide multiple large biopsy specimens for histologic evaluation and adjunctive procedures such as immunohistochemistry and electron microscopy [28–30]. It also provides information for staging, has prognostic value, and allows pleurodesis with agents such as talc. Early mesothelioma lesions are usually found on the lower parietal or diaphragmatic pleura and may resemble localized inflammation. The most typical lesions are rounded, more or less translucent masses (Figures 5.4 and 5.5), that vary in size from a pinhead to several centimeters. Irregular, bumpy infiltration or diffuse, difficult-to-biopsy pleural thickening may be seen (Figures 5.6 and 5.7). It may mimic metastatic tumor. There is no specific aspect for each histologic subtype of mesothelioma.

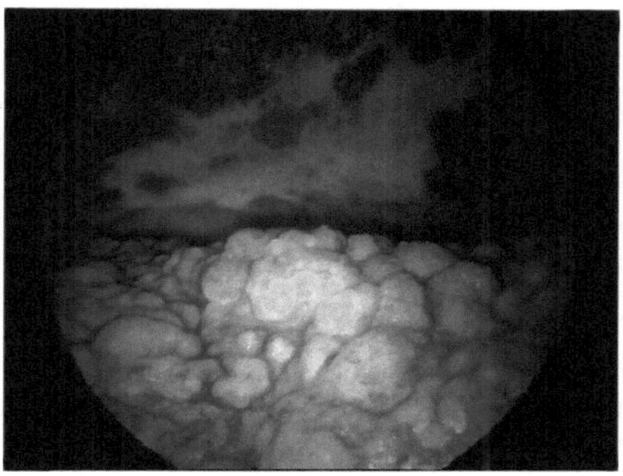

FIGURE 5.4. Thoracoscopic appearance of a diffuse nodular malignant mesothelioma (epithelioid).

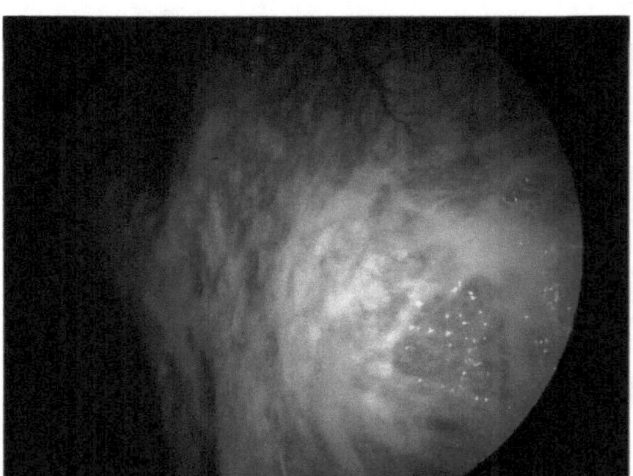

FIGURE 5.5. Thoracoscopic view of a diffuse malignant mesothelioma.

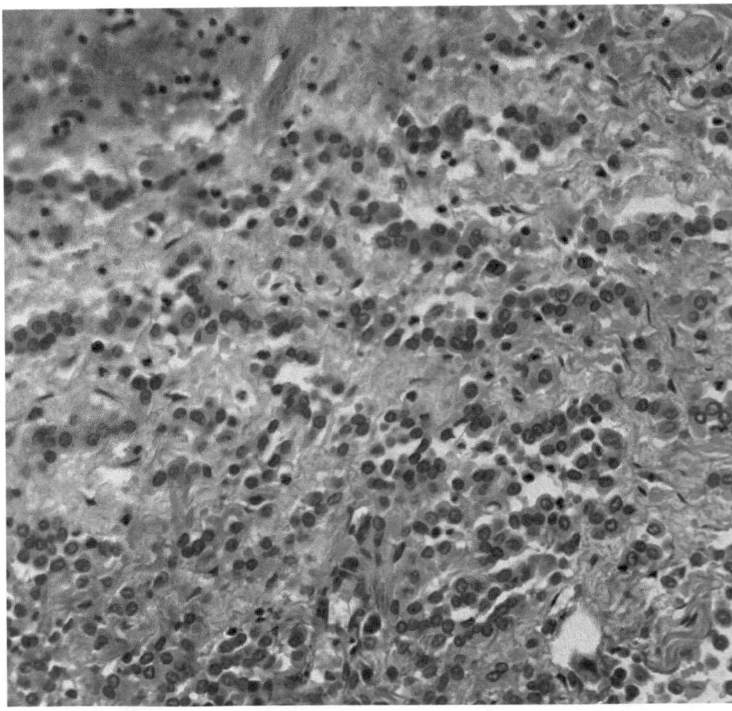

FIGURE 5.6. Thoracoscopic biopsy specimen from the same patient as Figure 5.5. It shows an epithelioid mesothelioma that infiltrated the parietal pleura in a single-file pattern.

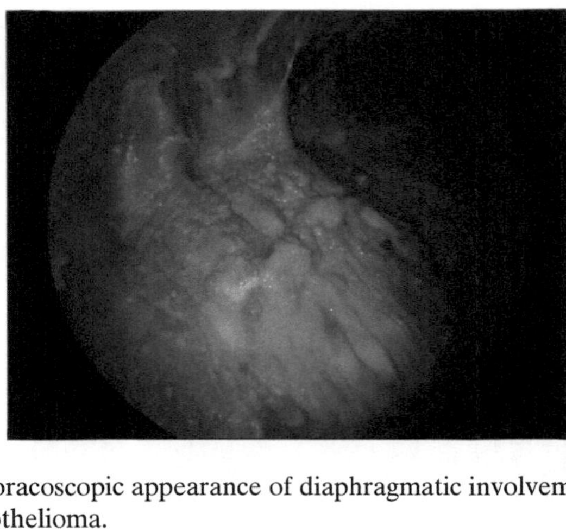

FIGURE 5.7. Thoracoscopic appearance of diaphragmatic involvement by a nodular malignant mesothelioma.

On the other hand, metastatic pleural malignancy usually shows scarce or numerous variable-sized tumor masses affecting mainly the parietal or diaphragmatic pleura (Figures 5.8–5.12) [31]. Diffuse infiltration and irregular thickening can also be seen. Sometimes candle wax-like lesions of the parietal pleura, which may be extensive, prove to be metastatic carcinoma. Even apparently inflammatory masses should be biopsied because they may prove to be malignant. All these tumoral masses of the parietal pleura may be hidden underneath a thick layer of fibrinous material and may need to be sought by deep biopsies.

The visceral pleura may also be affected although less frequently. A subpleural web is suggestive of carcinomatous lymphangitis. Peripheral pulmonary masses may occur and can be biopsied at thoracoscopy. Obviously,

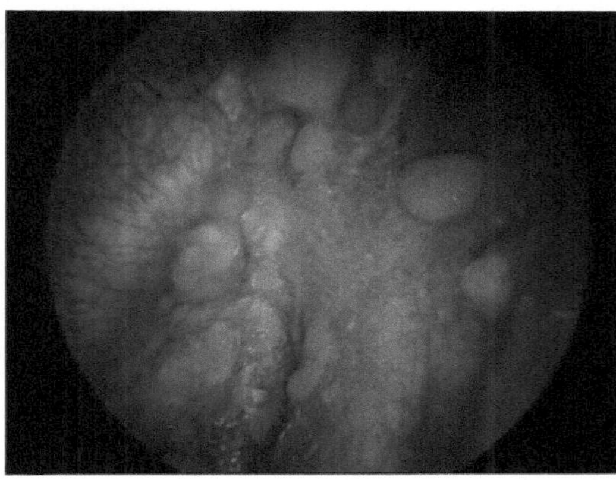

FIGURE 5.8. Discrete nodules from metastatic breast carcinoma.

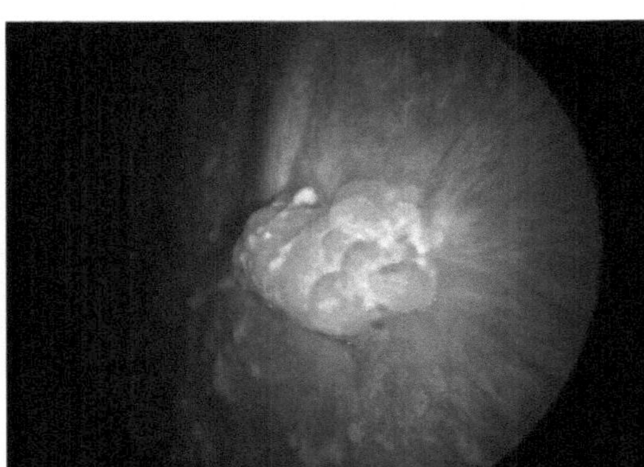

FIGURE 5.9. Large nodular mass with adjacent lymphangitic spread of tumor from a lung carcinoma.

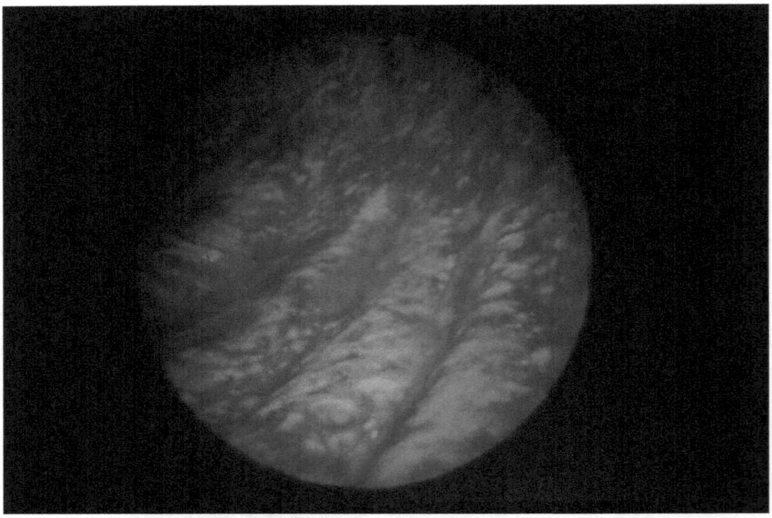

FIGURE 5.10. Tumor seedlings from a metastatic breast carcinoma.

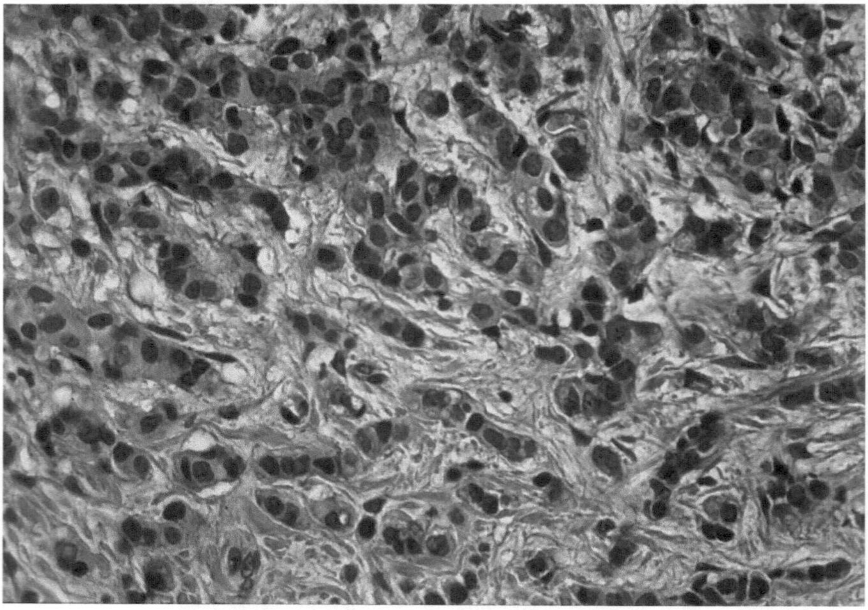

FIGURE 5.11. Thoracoscopic biopsy specimen from the same patient as in Figure 5.10, showing a metastatic breast carcinoma that infiltrated the pleura in a single file and that may be confused with diffuse epithelioid mesothelioma. The neoplastic cells were positive for estrogen receptor and negative for calretinin by immunohistochemistry.

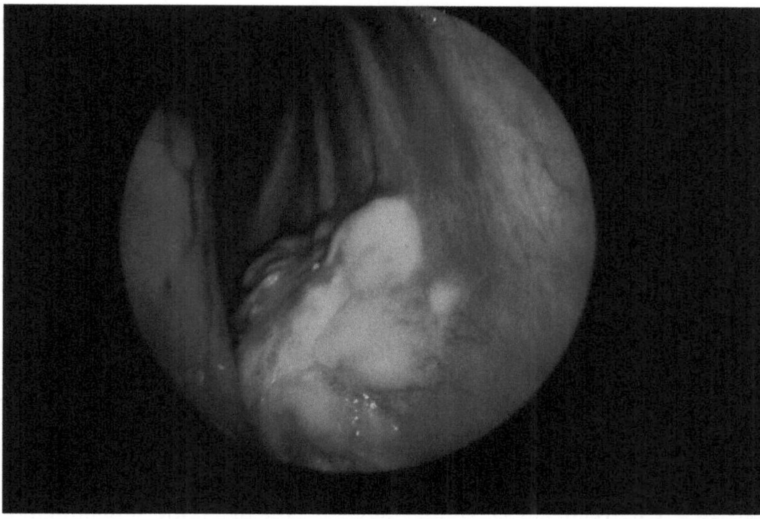

FIGURE 5.12. Thoracoscopic appearance of parietal involvement by a sarcoma.

such involvement of the visceral pleura cannot be detected by any closed (and therefore blind) needle biopsy.

Although a century-old procedure, thoracoscopy remains a highly valuable technique for exploring a pleural effusion when malignancy is suspected. It yields excellent diagnostic results and allows pleurodesis during the same procedure. Moreover, it is safe and does not require expensive equipment.

References

1. Maskell NA, Butland RJA. BTS guidelines for the investigation of a unilateral pleural effusion in adults. Thorax 2003;58(Suppl 2):8–17.
2. Sahn S. Pleural fluid analysis: narrowing the differential diagnosis. Semin Respir Med 1987;9:22–9.
3. Pettersson T, Froseth B, Riska H, et al. Concentration of hyaluronic acid in pleural fluid as a diagnostic aid for malignant mesothelioma. Chest 1988;94:1037–9.
4. Salyer WR, Eggleston JC, Erozan YS. Efficacy of pleural needle biopsy and pleural fluid cytopathology in the diagnosis of malignant neoplasm involving the pleura. Chest 1975;67:536–9.
5. Prakash UBS, Reiman HM. Comparison of needle biopsy with cytologic analysis for the evaluation of pleural effusions: analysis of 414 cases. Mayo Clin Proc 1985;60:158–64.
6. Whitaker D. The cytology of malignant mesothelioma. Cytopathology 2000;11:139–51.

7. McAleer JJ, Murphy GJ, Quinn RJ. Needle biopsy of the pleura in the diagnosis of pleural effusion. Ulster Med J 1987;56:54–7.
8. Loddenkemper R, Grosser H, Gabler A, et al. Prospective evaluation of biopsy methods in the diagnosis of malignant pleural effusions: intrapatient comparison between pleural fluid cytology, blind needle biopsy and thoracoscopy. Am Rev Respir Dis 1983;127(Suppl 4):114.
9. Poe RH, Israel RH, Utell MJ, et al. Sensitivity, specificity, and predictive values of closed pleural biopsy. Arch Intern Med 1984;144:325–8.
10. Walzl G, Wyser C, Smedema J, et al. Comparing the diagnostic yield of Abrams needle pleural biopsy and thoracoscopy. Am J Respir Crit Care Med 1996; 153:A460.
11. Kirsch CM, Kroe DM, Azzi RL, et al. The optimal number of pleural biopsy specimens for a diagnosis of tuberculous pleurisy. Chest 1997;112:702–6.
12. Emad A, Rezaian GR. Diagnostic value of closed percutaneous pleural biopsy vs pleuroscopy in suspected malignant pleural effusion or tuberculous pleurisy in a region with a high incidence of tuberculosis: a comparative, age-dependent study. Respir Med 1998;92:488–92.
13. Menzies R, Charbonneau M. Thoracoscopy for the diagnosis of pleural disease. Ann Intern Med 1991;114:271–6.
14. Kendall SW, Bryan AJ, Large SR, et al. Pleural effusions: is thoracoscopy a reliable investigation? A retrospective review. Respir Med 1992;86:437–40.
15. Loddenkemper R, Boutin C. Thoracoscopy: diagnostic and therapeutic indications. Eur Respir J 1993;6:1544–55.
16. Medical thoracoscopy: technique and indications in pulmonary medicine. J Bronchol 1994;1:228–39.
17. Harris RJ, Kavuru MS, Mehta AC, et al. The impact of thoracoscopy on the management of pleural disease. Chest 1995;107:845–52.
18. Harris RJ, Kavuru MS, Rice TW, et al. The diagnostic and therapeutic utility of thoracoscopy: a review. Chest 1995;108:828–41.
19. Loddenkemper R. Thoracoscopy—state of the art. Eur Respir J 1998;11: 213–21.
20. Blanc FX, Atassi K, Bignon J, et al. Diagnostic value of medical thoracoscopy in pleural disease. Chest 2002;121:1677–83.
21. Jacobaeus HC. Über die Möglichkeit, die Zystoskopie bei Untersuchung seröser Höhlen anzuwenden. Munch Med Wochenschr 1910;40:2090–2.
22. Jacobaeus HC. The cauterization of adhesions in artificial pneumothorax therapy of tuberculosis. Am Rev Tuberc 1922;6:871–97.
23. Aelony Y, King R, Boutin C. Thoracoscopic talc poudrage pleurodesis for chronic recurrent pleural effusions. Ann Intern Med 1991;115:778–82.
24. Mathur PN, Astoul P, Boutin C. Medical thoracoscopy: technical details. Clin Chest Med 1995;16:479–86.
25. Viskum K, Enk B. Complications of thoracoscopy. Poumon Cœur 1981;37:25–8.
26. Colt HG. Thoracoscopy: a prospective study of safety and outcome. Chest 1995;108:324–9.
27. Hansen M, Faurschou P, Clementsen P. Medical thoracoscopy, results and complications in 146 patients: a retrospective study. Respir Med 1998;92: 228–32.
28. Boutin C, Rey F. Thoracoscopy in pleural malignant mesothelioma: a prospective study of 188 consecutive patients. Part 1. Diagnosis. Cancer 1993;72:389–93.

29. Boutin C, Rey F, Gouvernet J, et al. Thoracoscopy in pleural malignant mesothelioma. Part 2. Prognosis and staging. Cancer 1993;72:394–404.
30. Boutin C, Schlesser M, Frenay C, et al. Malignant pleural mesothelioma. Eur Respir J 1998;12:972–81.
31. Boutin C, Viallat JR, Cargnino P, et al. Thoracoscopy in malignant pleural effusions. Am Rev Respir Dis 1981;124:588–92.

6
Pathologic Diagnosis and Classification of Mesothelioma

Cytologic specimens are often obtained in mesothelioma cases because of the high incidence of pleural effusion (Figure 6.1). A definitive diagnosis of mesothelioma based on cytologic specimens is controversial. This is due to the fact that when mesothelioma cells are sufficiently well differentiated to recognize their mesothelial nature, they are difficult to distinguish from reactive mesothelium. Similarly, when the cells are clearly malignant, it is difficult to distinguish mesothelioma cells from adenocarcinoma. Sarcomatoid mesotheliomas typically shed few tumor cells into the effusion (Figure 6.2). Some authorities diagnose a mesothelioma on a cytology specimen if sufficient numbers of cells are present in a cell block to permit ancillary histochemical, immunohistochemical, or ultrastructural studies (or a combination of these tests); others require the intact architecture obtained in a biopsy specimen before a definitive diagnosis is assigned [1–3]. Most panel members agree that a cytologic diagnosis of mesothelioma is possible provided appropriate clinical and radiologic features are present (Figures 6.3 and 6.4).

With approximately 50% of epithelioid mesotheliomas, the pleural fluid contains neoplastic cellular aggregates or individual neoplastic cells that may show solid aggregates or tubulopapillary features. In most cases in which cytologic evaluation is considered positive, there are numerous neoplastic cells. The immunohistochemical profile and the ultrastructural appearance of the cells in pleural fluid are the same as are seen in tissue specimens (Figure 6.5) [4–8]. When a sample of pleural fluid or ascitic fluid contains relatively few atypical cells consistent with mesothelial cells, caution should be used when making a diagnosis of epithelioid mesothelioma. As neoplastic cells in pleural or ascitic fluid become more anaplastic, it is more difficult to make a specific diagnosis.

With respect to fine-needle aspiration biopsy specimens, the same problems generally exist as with fluids; and whether a diagnosis can be made on a single specimen depends on the sample size and whether there are unequivocal malignant tissue/cells present. If unequivocal malignant tissue is present, immunohistochemical or ultrastrutural studies (or both) can be

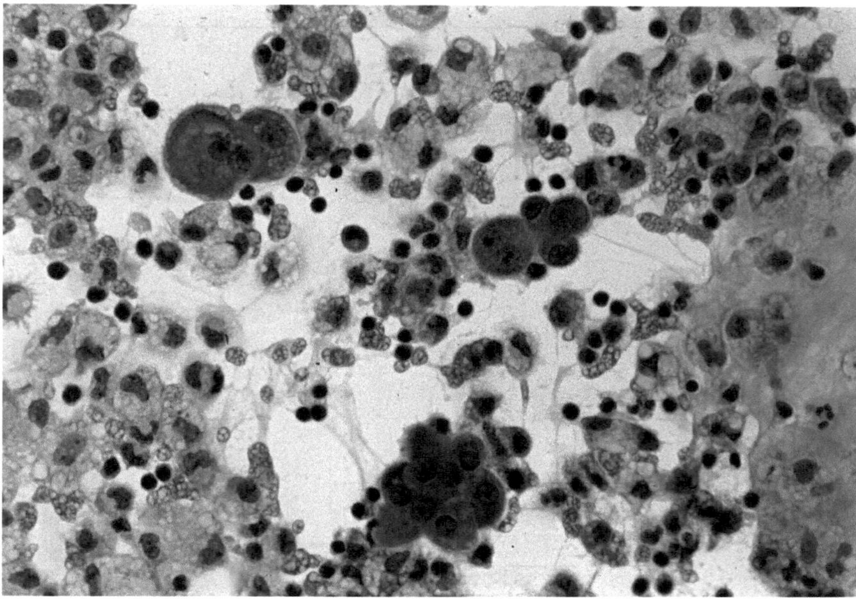

FIGURE 6.1. Papanicolaou stain from a cytologic preparation of a pleural effusion showing clusters of malignant mesothelial cells with central nuclei and small nucleoli. Note the high nuclear/cytoplasmic ratio and small peripheral submembranous vacuoles.

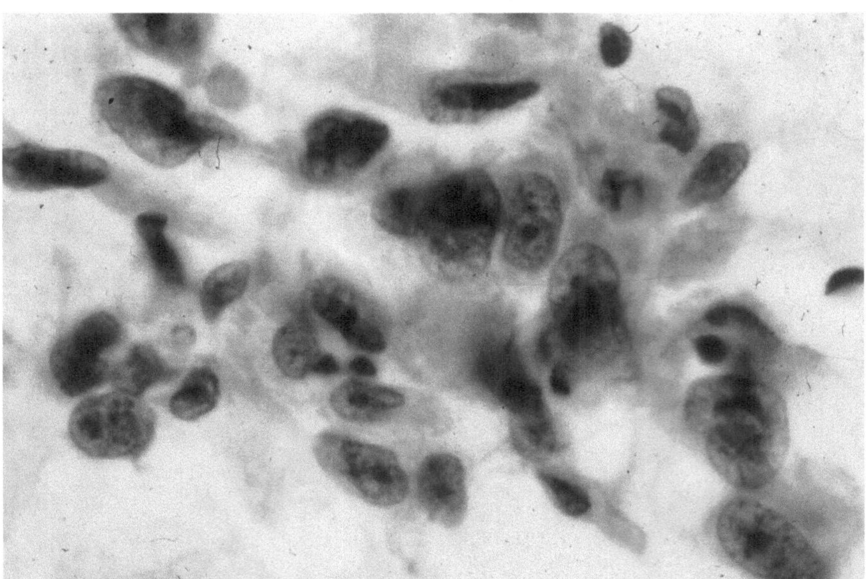

FIGURE 6.2. Papanicolaou stain from a fine-needle aspirate of a sarcomatoid pleural mesothelioma. The tumor metastasized to the spine and gingiva. Note the plump spindle cells with hyperchromatic nuclei and prominent nucleoli.

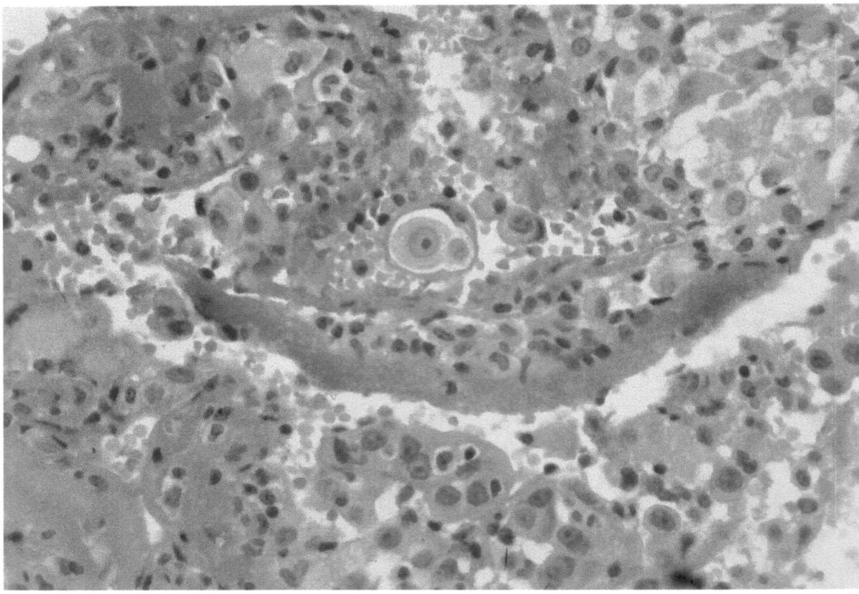

FIGURE 6.3. Cell block of a pleural effusion from a patient with a malignant epithelioid mesothelioma. Note the large epithelioid cells with central nuclei and small, centered nucleoli embedded in fibrin admixed with macrophages. Such specimens are difficult to distinguish from atypical reactive mesothelial cells.

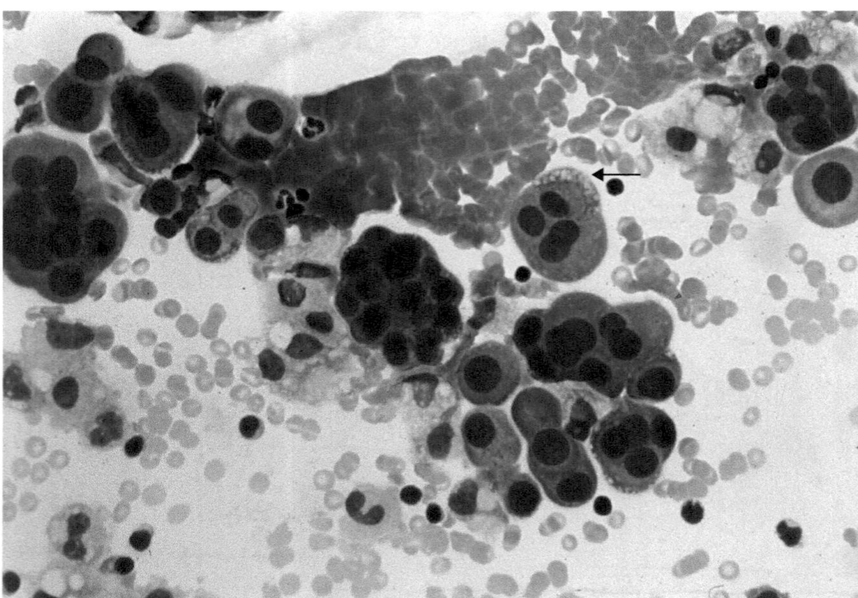

FIGURE 6.4. Cytologic preparation showing a cluster of neoplastic cells from a metastatic breast carcinoma admixed with reactive mesothelial cells showing small peripheral submembranous vacuoles.

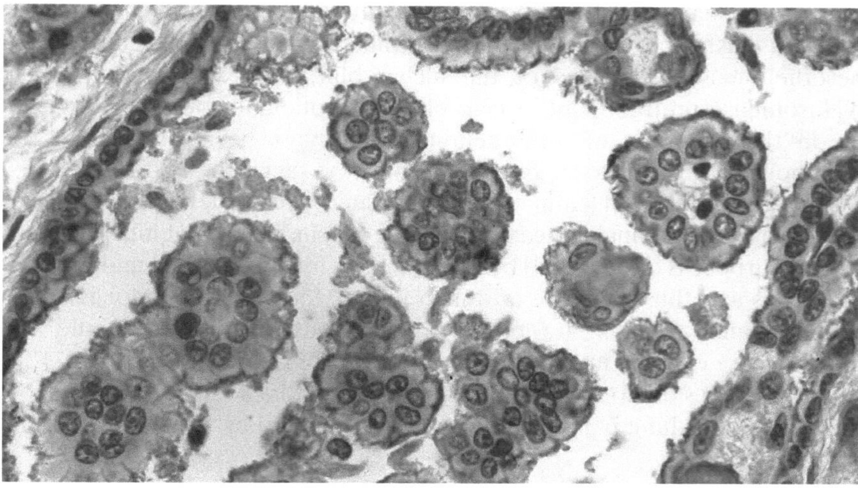

FIGURE 6.5. Cytologic specimen with a cluster of epithelioid malignant mesothelial cells showing strong membranous staining with HBME-1.

performed on the material to determine the nature of the neoplastic cells [2].

Pleural Biopsy

The diagnosis of mesothelioma and its distinction from other neoplasms and reactive processes with which it may be confused requires adequate tissue sampling. In most cases, this requires a thoracoscopic or open pleural biopsy specimen. If no tumor nodules are macroscopically visible and only diffuse pleural thickening is seen, it is advisable to take multiple *deep* biopsies of both the parietal and visceral pleura. In some cases, sufficient material is obtained from a core sample from a fine-needle aspirate to permit a firm diagnosis in conjunction with appropriate ancillary techniques (see below). Correlation of histopathologic studies or direct observation by the surgeon is important to avoid certain pitfalls in the diagnosis. A detailed protocol for the evaluation of pleural biopsy specimens has been described [9].

Histochemical Stains

Histochemical procedures can be useful for distinguishing epithelioid mesotheliomas from certain adenocarcinomas [7, 8]. The basis for this distinction is the detection of neutral mucins (produced in some adenocarcinomas) by means of the periodic acid-Schiff (PAS) stain following digestion with diastase, or the production of hyaluronic acid (produced by some mesotheliomas) by means of the alcian blue stain with and without hyaluronidase pretreatment. Alcian blue and colloidal iron are of limited use in the diagnosis of mesotheliomas and have been superceded by immunohistochemical techniques. Care must be taken to distinguish PAS-positive glycogen, basal lamina, and cytoplasmic glycoprotein globules from the spidery intraluminal appearance of true mucin. The use of mucicarmine for this purpose is discouraged because it stains hyaluronic acid under some conditions and thus gives the mistaken impression that the tumor is not a mesothelioma. Appropriate positive and negative controls should be applied. Rare cases of mucin-positive mesotheliomas are reported [10–12]. Asbestos bodies do not occur in pleura-based tumors, so iron stains are not indicated unless lung parenchyma has been obtained by the surgeon.

Immunohistochemistry

Immunohistochemical studies have grown in popularity during the past two decades and are frequently applied to distinguish mesothelioma from other neoplastic and reactive processes. Available methodology includes both the peroxidase-antiperoxidase method and the avidin biotinylated complex technique. A wide variety of immunohistochemical markers have been tested (see Table 8.1), and their utility in various diagnostic circumstances is detailed below (Figures 6.5 and 6.6). No single immunohistochemical marker is diagnostic of, or absolutely excludes, mesothelioma, so panels of markers are recommended to distinguish mesothelioma from other malignant or reactive processes. The panel used must be tailored to the diagnostic circumstances. A differential diagnosis should be generated based on the appearance of the lesion on hematoxylin and eosin-stained sections, and the immunohistochemical panel selected should be suitable to sort out the various diagnostic possibilites. Appropriate positive and negative controls should always be applied.

Electron Microscopy

Ultrastructurally, it is not possible to differentiate neoplastic from reactive mesothelial cells reliably. Ultrastructural studies, however, are useful for distinguishing mesothelioma from carcinoma, and this procedure can be both rapid and cost-effective compared with other ancillary techniques [4, 7, 13]. Electron microscopy is most helpful in the setting of conflicting immunohistochemical staining results. Glutaraldehyde fixation is optimal, but 10% buffered formalin works almost as well. The key feature is to be sure that the tissue sample is thin enough to allow adequate pene-

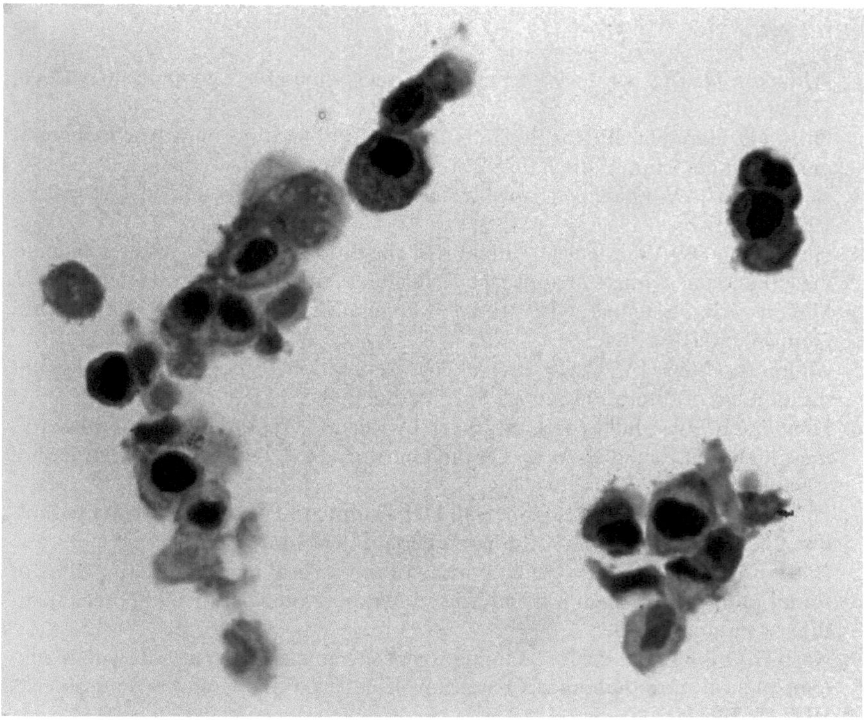

FIGURE 6.6. Cytologic preparation showing nuclear staining with calretinin in a malignant epithelioid mesothelioma.

tration of the fixative solution. In fact, most of the ultrastructural features that aid in distinguishing mesothelioma from other conditions are preserved in paraffin-embedded tissues, and retrieval from paraffin can provide useful information when glutaraldehyde or formalin-fixed wet tissue is no longer available.

Other Special Techniques

It is possible that in situ hybridization and other molecular techniques will prove useful in the future pathologic diagnosis of mesothelioma. Some studies require frozen tissue specimens, but those that gain the widest acceptance and usage will be the ones that work on paraffin-embedded specimens. For many tumors, specific genetic markers have been identified that may assist in the diagnosis. Although no such marker is currently available for mesothelioma, it is likely that such a genetic marker will be forthcoming. Comparison with established ancillary techniques are necessary to establish the utility of such novel diagnostic approaches [14–17].

References

1. Whitaker D. The cytology of malignant mesothelioma. Cytopathology 2000; 11:139–51.
2. Oury TD, Hammar SP, Roggli VL. Ultrastructural features of diffuse malignant mesothelioma. Hum Pathol 1998;29:1382–92.
3. Bedrossian CW. Diagnostic problems in serous effusions. Diagn Cytopathol 1998;19:131–7.
4. Henderson DW, Whitaker D, Shilkin KB. The differential diagnosis of malignant mesothelioma: a practical approach to diagnosis during life. In: Henderson DW, Shilkin KB, Langlois SLP (eds) Malignant mesothelioma. New York: Hemisphere; 1992:184.
5. Churg A, Colby TV, Cagle P, et al. The separation of benign and malignant mesothelial proliferations. Am J Surg Pathol 2000;24:1183–200.
6. Henderson DW, Shilkin KB, Whitaker D. Reactive mesothelial hyperplasia vs mesothelioma, including mesothelioma in situ: a brief review. Am J Clin Pathol 1998;110:397–404.
7. Hammar SP. Pleural diseases. In: Dail DH, Hammar SP (eds) Pulmonary pathology, 2nd edition. New York: Springer-Verlag; 1994:1463–579.
8. Battifora H, McCaughey WTE. Tumors of the serosal membranes. In: Atlas of tumor pathology, 3rd edition. Fascicle 15. Washington, DC: Armed Forces Institute of Pathology; 1995.
9. Nash G, Otis C. Protocol for examination of specimens from patients with malignant pleural mesothelioma: a basis for checklists. Canc Coll Am Pathologists 1999;123:39–44.
10. Hammar SP, Bockus DE, Remington FL, et al. Mucin-positive epithelial mesotheliomas: a histochemical, immunohistochemical and ultrastructural comparison with mucin-producing pulmonary adenocarcinomas. Ultrastructural pathology 1996;20:293–325.
11. Robb JA. Mesothelioma versus adenocarcinoma: false positive CEA and LeuM1 staining due to hyaluronic acid. Hum Pathol 1989;20:400.
12. Cook DS, Attanoos RK, Jalloh SS, et al. 'Mucin positive' epithelial mesothelioma of the peritoneum: an unusual diagnostic pitfall. Histopathology 2000; 17:33–6.
13. Ordonez NG, Mackay B. The roles of immunohistochemistry and electron microscopy in distinguishing epithelial mesothelioma of the pleura from adenocarcinoma. Adv Anat Pathol 1996;3:273–93.
14. Lugli A, Forster Y, Haas P, et al. Calretinin expression in human normal and neoplastic tissues: a tissue microarray analysis on 5233 tissue samples. Hum Pathol 2003;34:994–1000.
15. Puntoni R, Filiberti R, Cerrano PG, et al. Implementation of a molecular epidemiology approach to human pleural malignant mesothelioma. Mutat Res 2003;544:385–96.
16. Segers K, Ramael M, Singh SK, et al. Detection of numerical chromosomal aberrations in paraffin-embedded malignant pleural mesothelioma by non-isotopic in situ hybridization. J Pathol 1995;175:219–26.
17. Zimmerman RL, Bibbo M. Clinical utility of chromosome 17 alpha satellite probe in distinguishing benign mesothelium from malignant cells: a pilot study using routinely fixed specimens. Oncol Rep 1999;6:695–8.

7
Macroscopic Features of Mesotheliomas

The macroscopic appearance of a mesothelioma [1] depends on when in its natural history the mesothelioma is first observed. In individuals who present acutely with effusions, it is not uncommon on thoracoscopic or laparoscopic evaluation to see the visceral and parietal layers of the serosal membrane studded by multiple, usually small nodules of tumor (Figure 7.1a). As pleural mesotheliomas progress, the individual nodules presumably coalesce to form a rind of tumor that encases the lung (Figures 7.1b, 7.2, 7.3). Typically, they grow along the interlobar fissures with little lung parenchymal involvement (Figure 7.4). Approximately one-third of pleural mesotheliomas directly invade the parietal pericardium and sometimes the visceral pericardium (Figures 7.5 and 7.6). Rarely, mesotheliomas invade most of the pericardium and sometimes extensively infiltrate the myocardium. In some instances, mesotheliomas present as mediastinal or hilar masses, which usually are due to enlarged lymph nodes involved by metastatic mesothelioma (Figures 7.7 through 7.9). Rarely, patients have been seen with a pleural mesothelioma in which the pleural tumor was not thick enough to be observed radiographically but a localized mass was observed in the lung or mediastinum [2]. Mesotheliomas not infrequently have a nodular appearance on their external surface and directly invade the lung parenchyma, producing large nodular masses. Masses in the lung parenchyma are often more obvious radiographically than thickened pleura and can be misinterpreted as primary lung neoplasms. Most mesotheliomas are thicker at the base of the lung than they are at the apex. Variation in the thickness of the ring of mesothelioma encasing the lung is common, and occasionally there is separate involvement of visceral and parietal pleura by tumor (Figure 7.10).

Mesotheliomas commonly metastasize [3]. The most frequent site of metastases for pleural mesothelioma is through lymphatics to bronchopulmonary, hilar, and mediastinal lymph nodes; occasionally, lymphangitic spread is observed. The next most frequent site of metastasis is the visceral pleural surface of the contralateral lung (Figure 7.11). Pleural mesotheliomas may directly invade through the diaphragm into the peritoneal

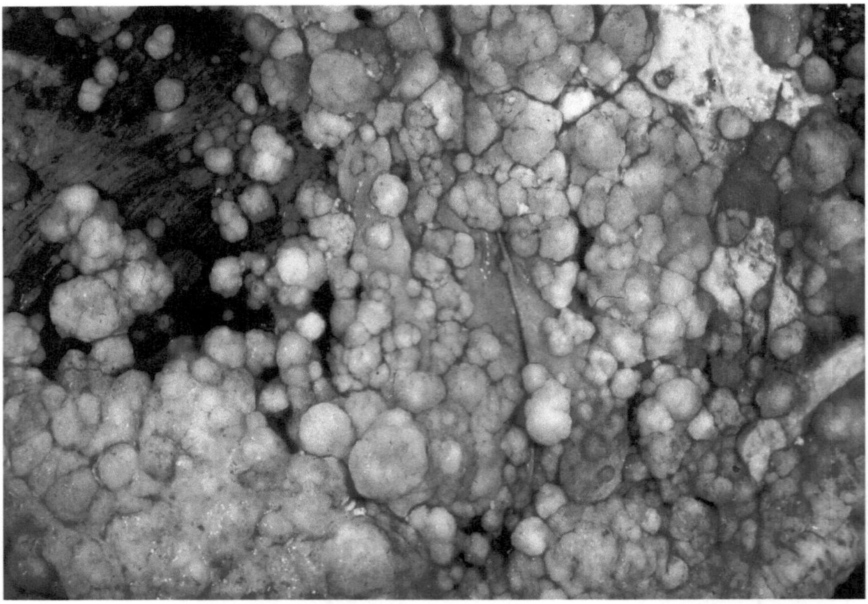

A

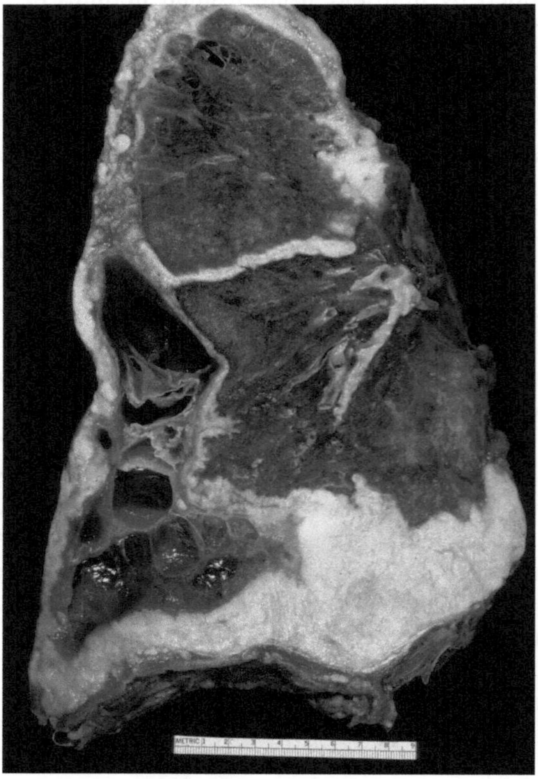

B

FIGURE 7.1. A. Visceral layer of the serosal membrane studded by multiple, small nodules of tumor. B. Example of diffuse malignant pleural mesothelioma. The tumor typically forms a rind around the lung and obliterates the pleural cavity. Variation in thickness of the rind of mesothelioma is common, usually being thicker at the base than the apex. Occasionally, there is separation of involved parietal and visceral pleura.

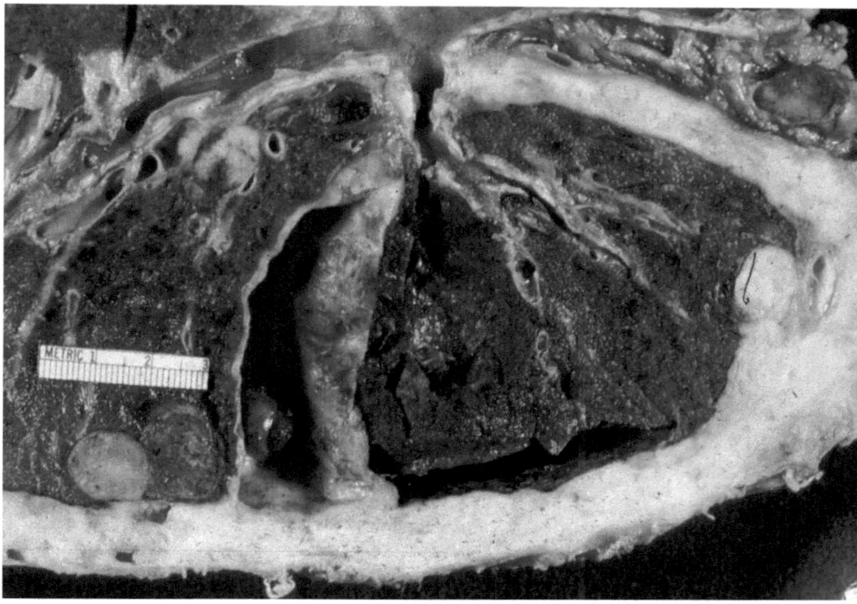

FIGURE 7.2. Mesotheliomas frequently have a nodular external surface and directly invade lung parenchyma.

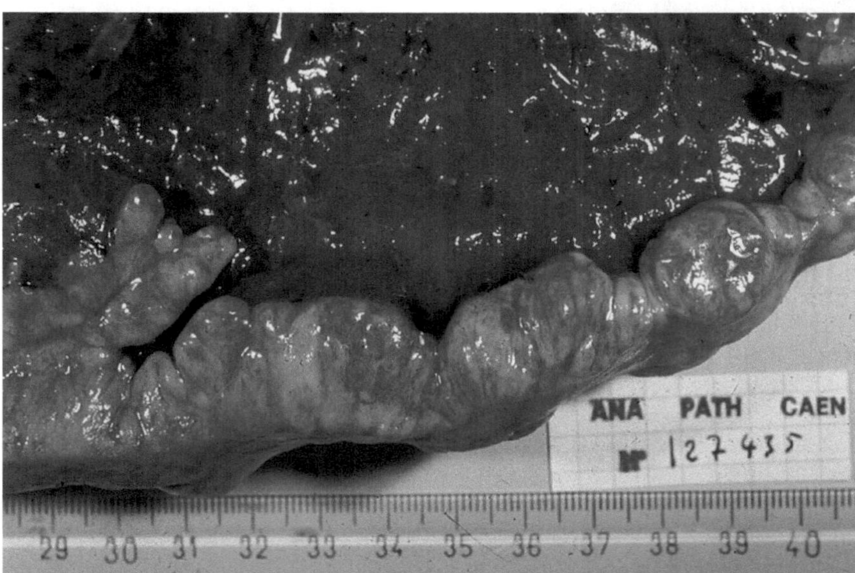

FIGURE 7.3. Mesothelioma showing diffuse involvement of the visceral pleura.

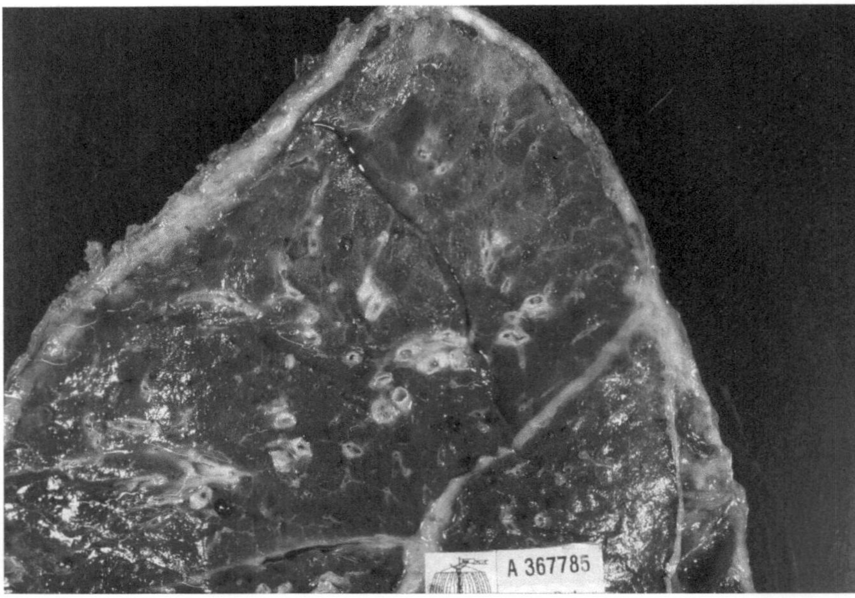

FIGURE 7.4. Diffuse pleural mesothelioma involving interlobar fissure with little lung parenchymal involvement.

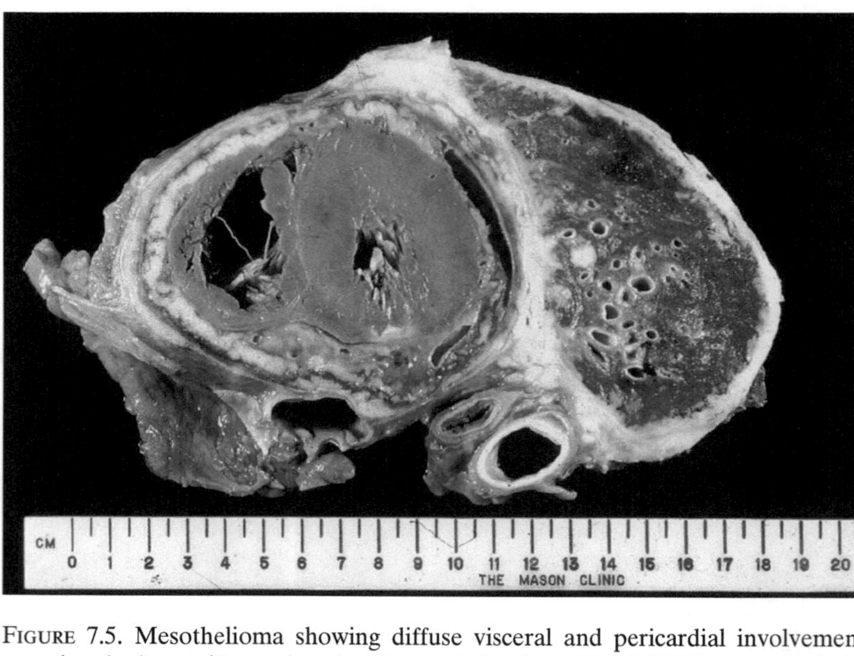

FIGURE 7.5. Mesothelioma showing diffuse visceral and pericardial involvement encasing the heart. (Reporduced with permission from Dail DH, Hammar SP [eds] Dail and Hammar's pulmonary pathology, 2nd edition. Vol 1: Non-neoplastic. New York: Springer-Verlag New York, 1994:1496.)

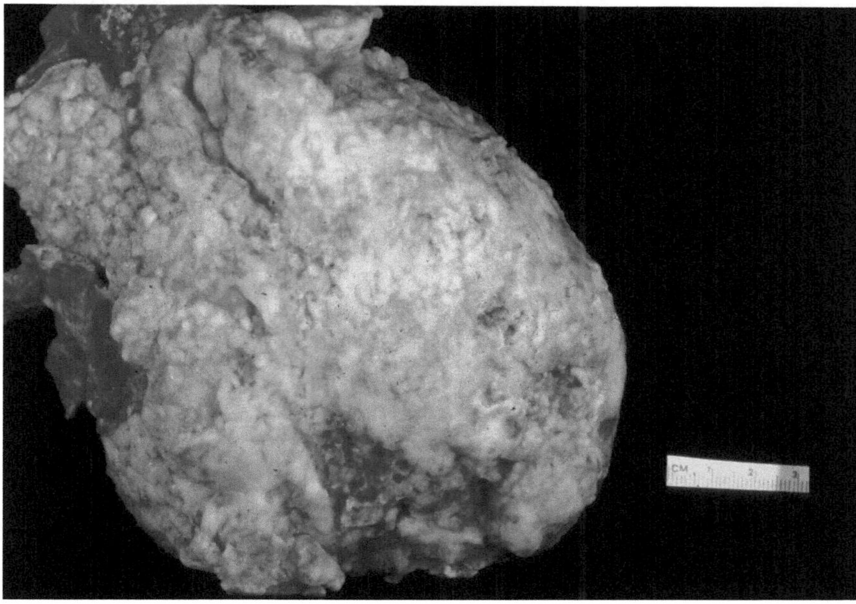

FIGURE 7.6. Mesothelioma showing diffuse pericardial involvement.

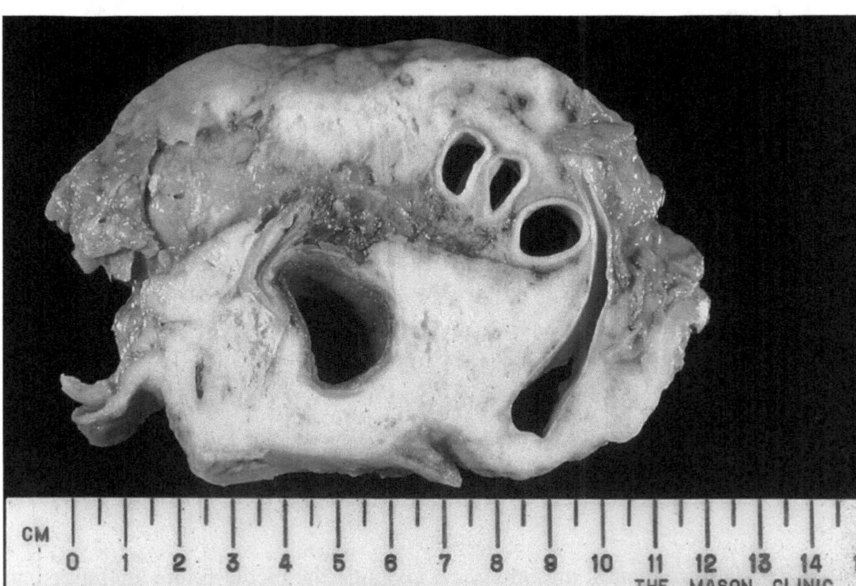

FIGURE 7.7. Mediastinal involvement by mesothelioma.

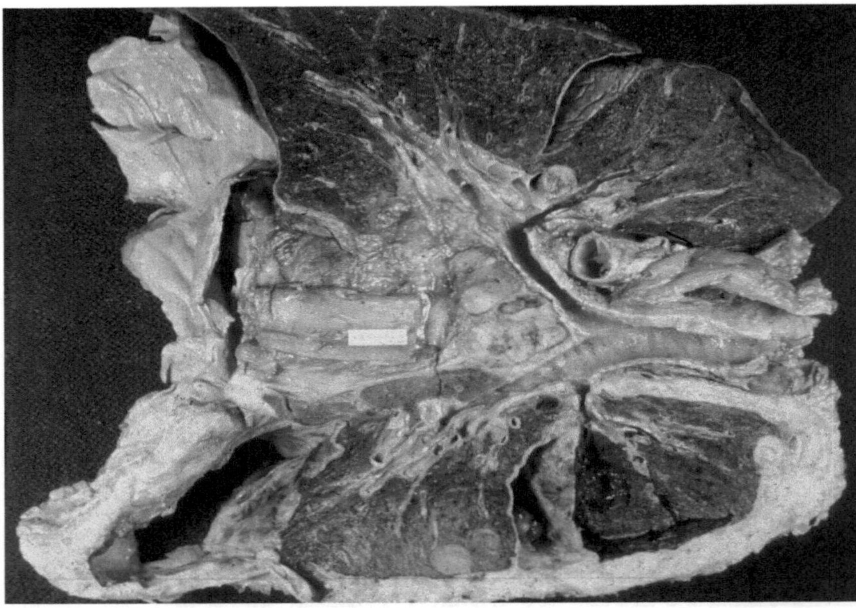

FIGURE 7.8. Diffuse mesothelioma showing mediastinal lymph node involvement.

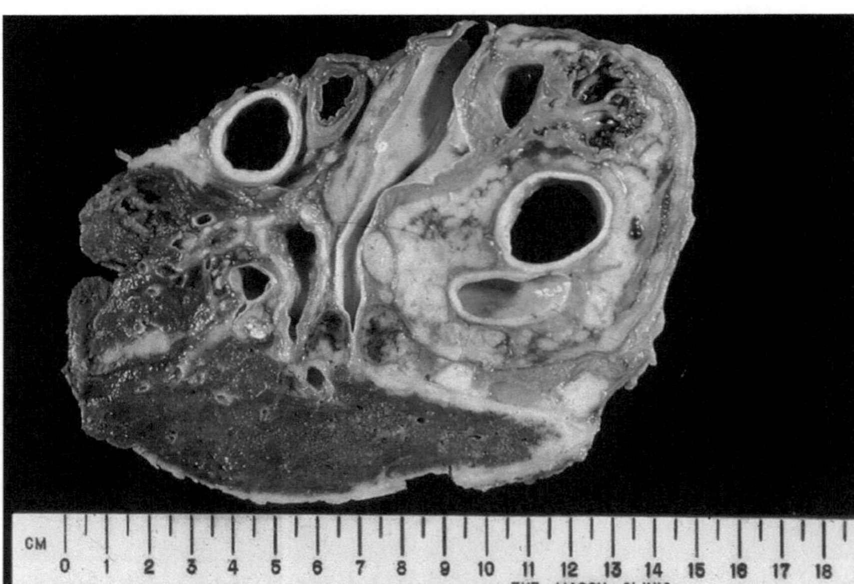

FIGURE 7.9. Diffuse pleural mesothelioma invading the mediastinum and encasing the great vessels.

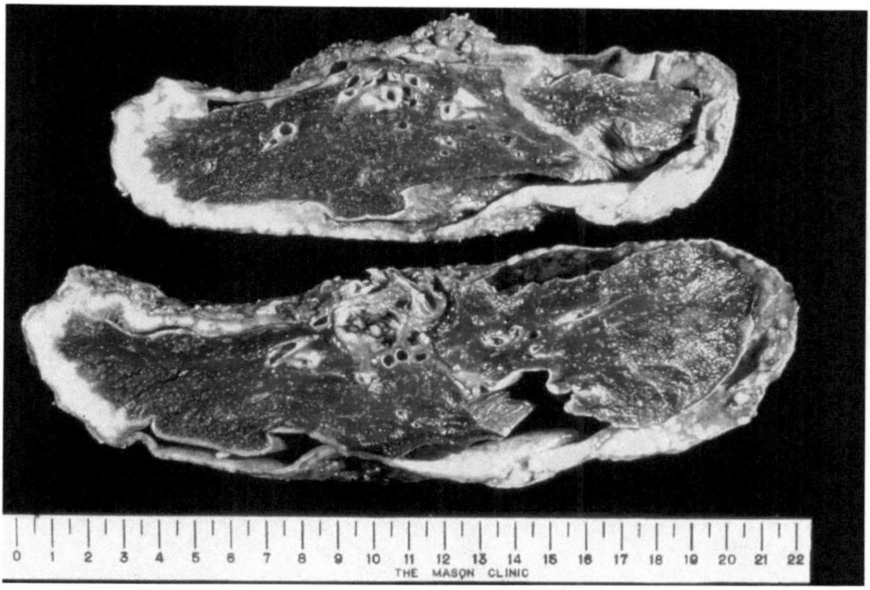

FIGURE 7.10. Diffuse pleural mesothelioma with encasement of the lung showing variation in the thickness of the ring of mesothelioma with separate involvement of the visceral and parietal pleura.

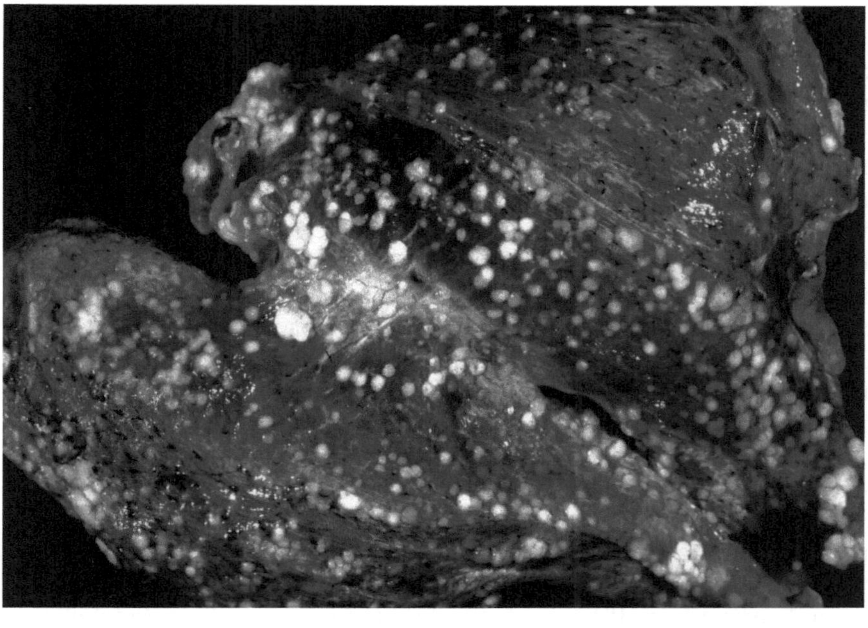

FIGURE 7.11. Diffuse pleural mesothelioma showing small metastatic nodules in the contralateral visceral pleura.

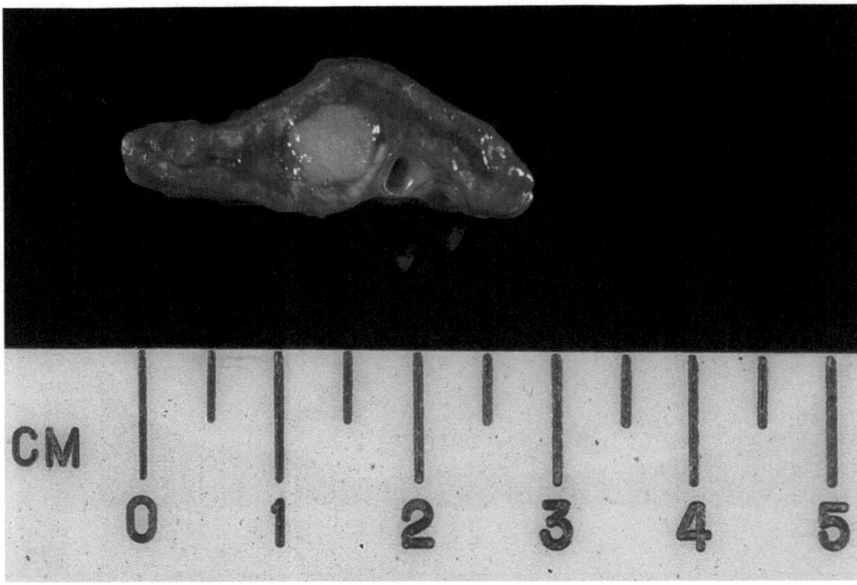

FIGURE 7.12. Adrenal gland showing a metastasis from a pleural mesothelioma. (Reproduced with permission from Dail DH, Hammar SP [eds] Dail and Hammar's pulmonary pathology, 2nd edition. Vol 1: Non-neoplastic. New York: Springer-Verlag New York, 1994:1501.)

cavity. Mesotheliomas can metastasize to brain, bone, liver, and adrenal glands (Figure 7.12) and to other serosal surfaces, especially peritoneum in the case of pleural mesotheliomas. Epithelioid mesotheliomas that produce excessive amounts of hyaluronic acid or proteoglycans are not uncommon and are characteristically "slimy." During sectioning, they may be extremely difficult to grasp because of the "slimy" characteristic of the proteoglycans and hyaluronic acid. Mesotheliomas that produce excessive amounts of hyaluronic acid/proteoglycans usually form varying thin-walled, translucent cysts in the tumor that are filled with the secretory product (Figure 7.13). Desmoplastic malignant mesothelioma in most cases cannot be differentiated from diffuse fibrous pleuritis macroscopically. Rarely, mesotheliomas mimic sclerosing mediastinitis grossly.

Hyaline pleural plaques may be observed in those with asbestos exposure and are commonly found to be associated with mesotheliomas [4]. Plaques are observed most frequently on the diaphragmatic parietal pleura and the lateral chest wall (Figure 7.14), usually in the distribution of the ribs. Plaques are rarely seen on the visceral pleura covering the lung and visceral pericardium. Plaques identical to those seen on the parietal pleura have been observed in the abdominal cavity, most frequently on the splenic surface. Sometimes plaques are discovered on histology.

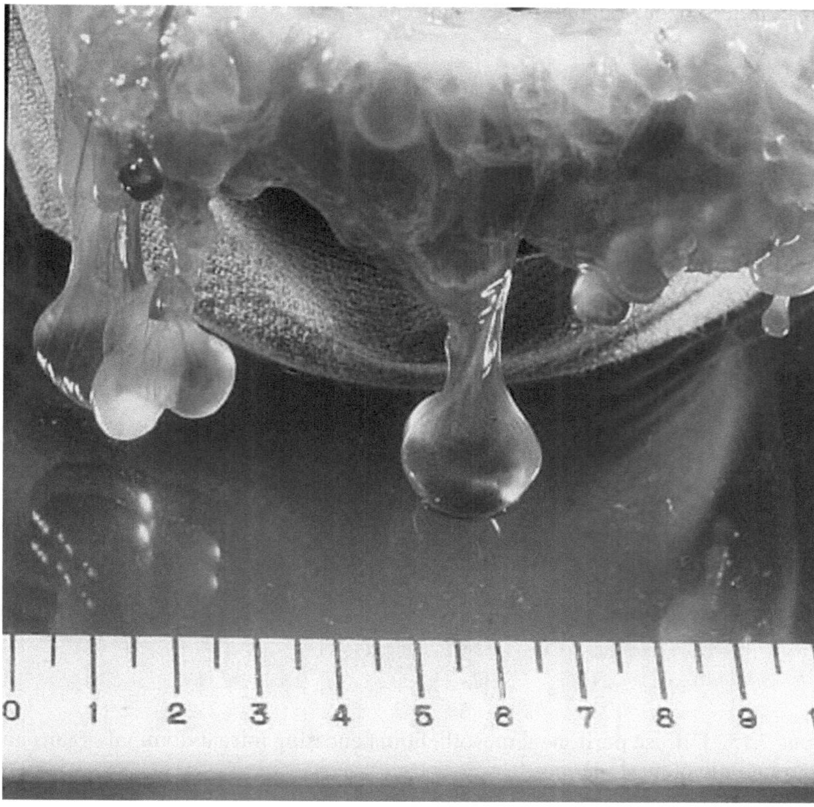

FIGURE 7.13. Globules of hyaluronic acid exuding from a pleural mesothelioma.

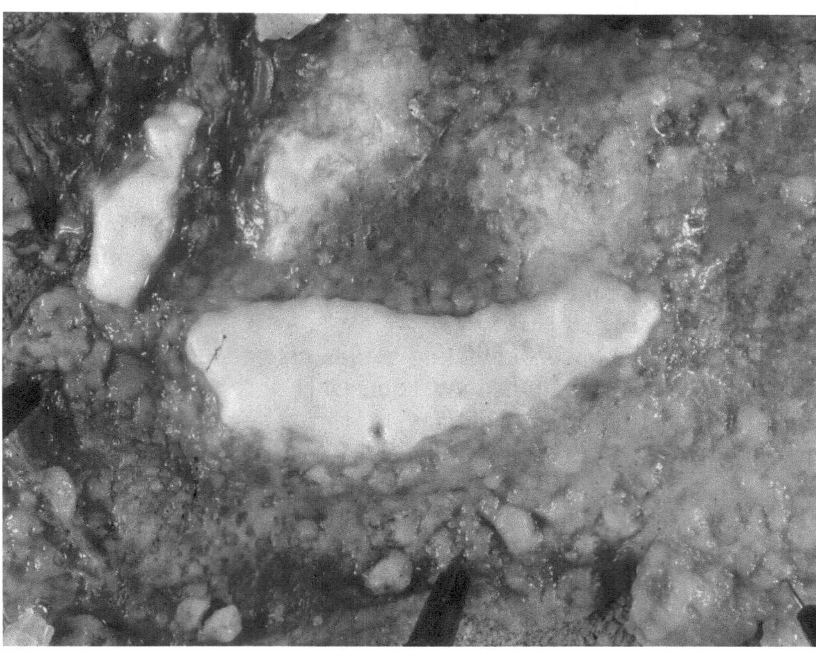

FIGURE 7.14. Retrosternal pleural plaques associated with diffuse pleural mesothelioma.

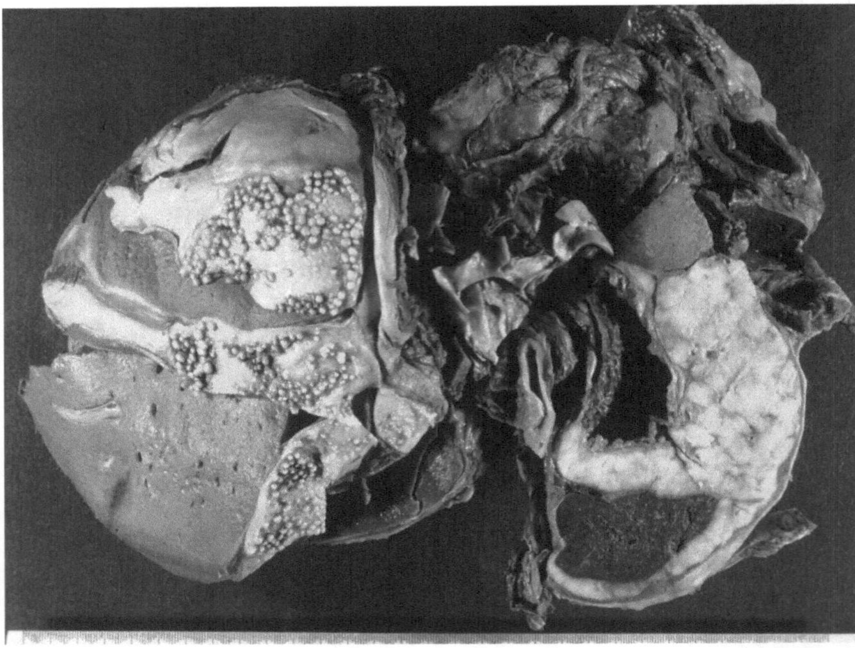

FIGURE 7.15. Diffuse peritoneal mesothelioma encasing intraabdominal organs and diaphragmatic pleural plaques.

At initial evaluation, peritoneal mesotheliomas often consist of multiple small nodules studding the visceral and parietal peritoneum [5]. As peritoneal mesotheliomas grow, they progressively encase organs in the abdominal cavity (Figure 7.15). In contrast, well-differentiated papillary epithelioid mesothelioma of the peritoneum, an uncommon mesothelial proliferation, is characterized by small nodules less than 1 cm that spread over the peritoneal surface of abdominal organs. It is macroscopically distinct from conventional diffuse malignant mesotheliomas, which are usually larger and more diffuse. Peritoneal cysts are characterized by multiple small, thin-walled, translucent cysts; and they have to be differentiated from malignant mesotheliomas, which sometimes form large cysts because they are reactive lesions [5–10].

Ovarian mesotheliomas simulating serous carcinomas and multicystic mesotheliomas, were mentioned in Chapter 4 [11].

Primary pericardial mesotheliomas are rare. They grow like mesotheliomas in other sites and encase the heart.

The tunica vaginalis is a recognized primary site of mesotheliomas. Mesotheliomas that arise in this location characteristically have the same histologic features of mesotheliomas that arise in the peritoneal cavity and pleural cavities [12]. They usually present as a nodule in this anatomic site.

Solitary well-differentiated papillary mesotheliomas may also be observed in this site [13, 14].

References

1. Churg A. Neoplastic asbestos induced disease. In: Churg A, Green FHY (eds) Pathology of occupational lung disease, 2nd edition. Baltimore: Williams & Wilkins; 1998:356.
2. Crotty TB, Myers JL, Katzenstein AL, et al. Localized malignant mesothelioma: a clinicopathologic and flow cytometric study. Am J Surg Pathol 1994;18:357–63.
3. King JA, Tucker JA, Wong SW. Mesothelioma: a study of 22 cases. South Med J 1997;90:199–205s.
4. Roggli VL, Sharma A, Butnor KJ, et al. Malignant mesothelioma and occupational exposure to asbestos: a clinicopathological correlation of 1445 cases. Ultrastruct Pathol 2002;26:55–65.
5. Daya D, McCaughey. Pathology of the peritoneum: a review of selected topics. Semin Diagn Pathol 1991;8:277–89.
6. Goldblum J, Hart WR. Localized and diffuse mesotheliomas of the genital tract and peritoneum in women: a clinicopathologic study of nineteen true mesothelial neoplasms, other than adenomatoid tumors, multicystic mesotheliomas, and localized fibrous tumors. Am J Surg Pathol 1995;19:1124–37.
7. Galateau-Salle F, Vignaud JM, Burke L, et al. Well differentiated papillary mesothelioma of the pleura: a series of 24 cases. Am J Surg Pathol 2004; 28:534–40.
8. Butnor KJ, Sporn TA, Hammar SP, et al. Well–differentiated papillary mesothelioma. Am J Surg Pathol 2001;10:1304–9.
9. Foyle A, Al-jabi M, McCaughey WT. Papillary peritoneal tumors in women. Am J Surg Pathol 1981:5;241–9.
10. Daya D, McCaughey. Well differentiated papillary mesothelioma of the peritoneum. Cancer 1990;65:292–6.
11. Gilks CB, Bell DA, Scully RE. Serous psammocarcinoma of the ovary and peritoneum. Int J Gynaecol Pathol 1990;9:110–21.
12. Jones A, Young RH, Scully RE. Malignant mesothelioma of the tunica vaginalis: a clinicopathologic analysis of 11 cases with review of the literature. Am J Surg Pathol 1995;7:815–25.
13. Barbera V, Rubino M. Papillary mesothelioma of the tunica vaginalis. Cancer 1957;10:182–9.
14. Xiao SY, Rizzo P, Carbone M. Benign papillary mesothelioma of the tunica vaginalis testis. Arch Pathol Lab Med 2000;124:143–7.

8 Classification and Histologic Features of Mesotheliomas

According to the 2004 World Health Organization (WHO) classification there are three major histologic subtypes of malignant mesothelioma: epithelioid, sarcomatoid (including desmoplastic) and biphasic [1]. Within these subtypes there are myriad patterns, of which it is important to be aware in terms of the histopathologic diagnosis, although they are not significant clinically [2–5].

Epithelioid Mesothelioma

Epithelioid or epithelial malignant mesotheliomas consist of tubules, acini, papillae, or sheets of atypical, epithelioid mesothelial cells. Like primary pulmonary adenocarcinomas, epithelioid mesotheliomas show a wide range of differentiation, and it is common to see several histologic patterns in most epithelioid mesotheliomas. Tubulopapillary epithelioid mesotheliomas are formed by small to medium-sized cuboidal cells with fairly uniform, round nuclei that have small to medium-sized nucleoli (Figures 8.1 and 8.2). The papillary structures usually have fibrovascular cores. Most tubulopapillary epithelioid mesotheliomas are well differentiated, although they can be formed by anaplastic cells. Psammoma bodies are occasionally seen in tubulopapillary mesotheliomas but not as frequently as in some papillary carcinomas (e.g., serous papillary carcinoma of the peritoneum) (Figure 8.3). Glandular (adenomatoid) mesotheliomas (Figures 8.4 and 8.5) may be confused with primary pulmonary adenocarcinomas or metastatic acinar adenocarcinomas. Occasionally, some epithelioid mesotheliomas are formed by large columnar mesothelial cells (Figure 8.6) and closely resemble pulmonary adenocarcinoma. Mesotheliomas may show solid sheets (Figure 8.7) of polygonal cells that resemble large cell carcinoma (Figure 8.8). Histiocytoid mesotheliomas are composed of cells that resemble pulmonary alveolar macrophages (Figure 8.9).

There is a spectrum of differentiation, from a solid mesothelioma to a type of mesothelioma referred to as "deciduoid" mesothelioma in which the

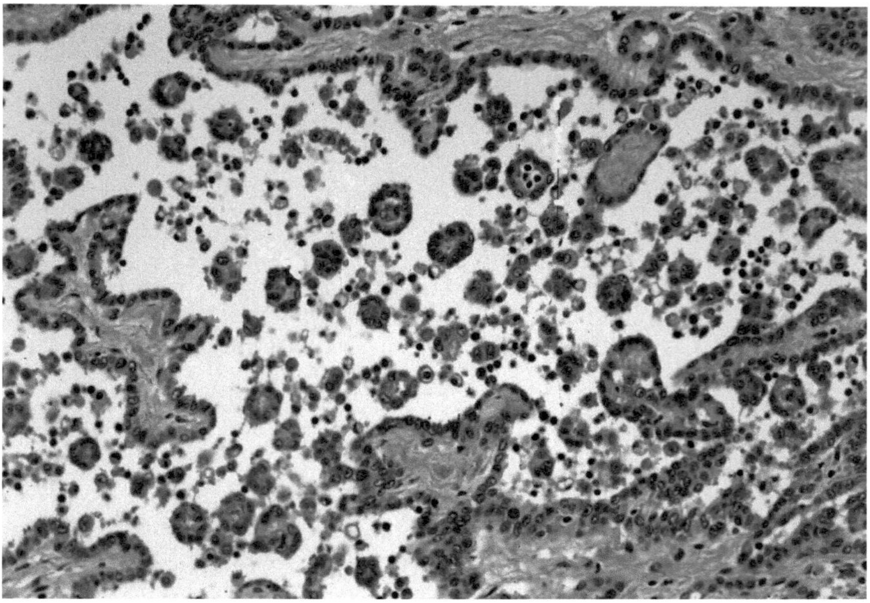

FIGURE 8.1. Malignant mesothelioma showing tubulopapillary differentiation.

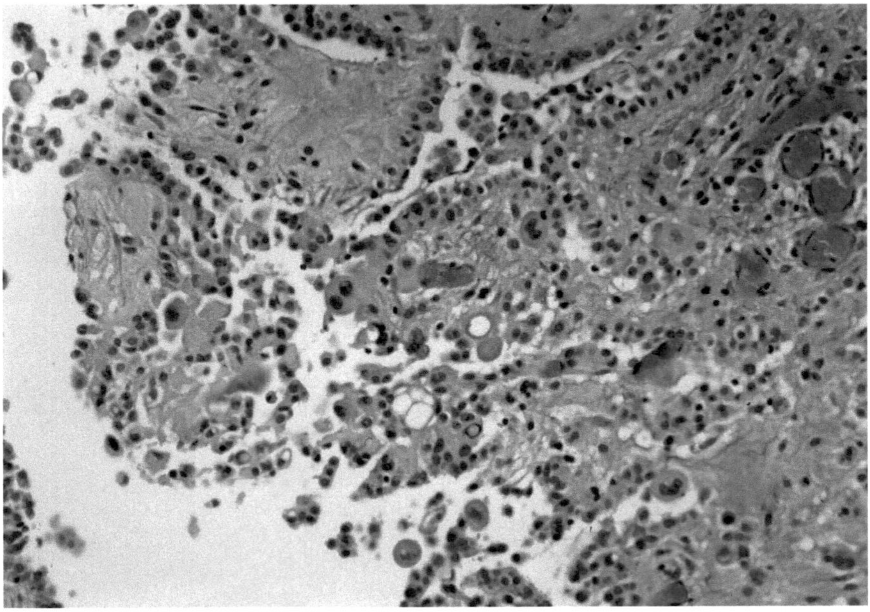

FIGURE 8.2. Malignant mesothelioma with tubules and papillae containing fibrous cores and epithelioid cells infiltrating the cores.

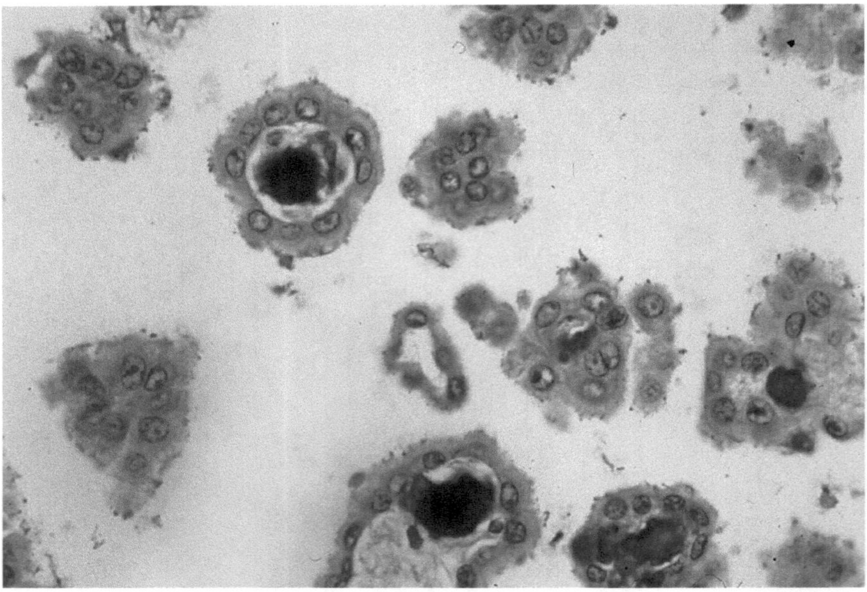

Figure 8.3. Mesothelioma with papillae and psammomas bodies.

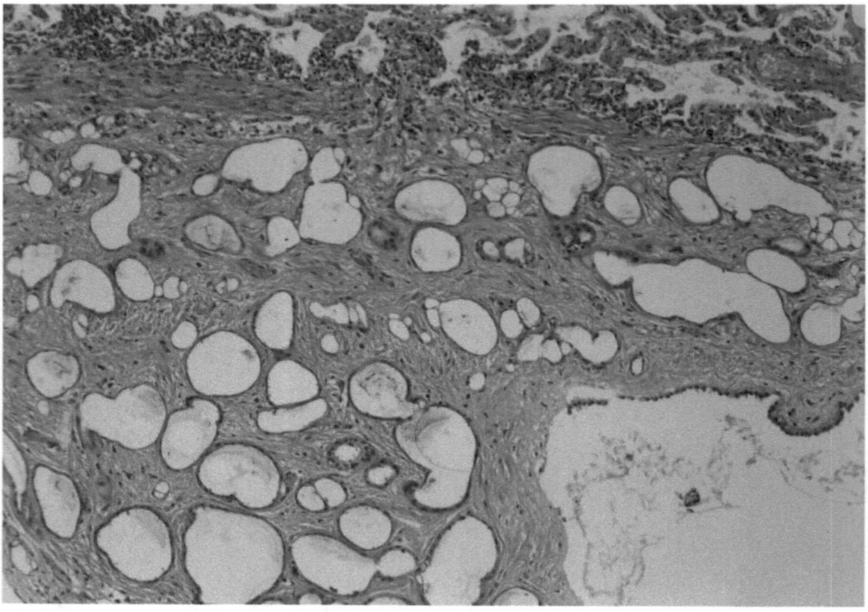

Figure 8.4. Mesothelioma showing adenomatoid pattern.

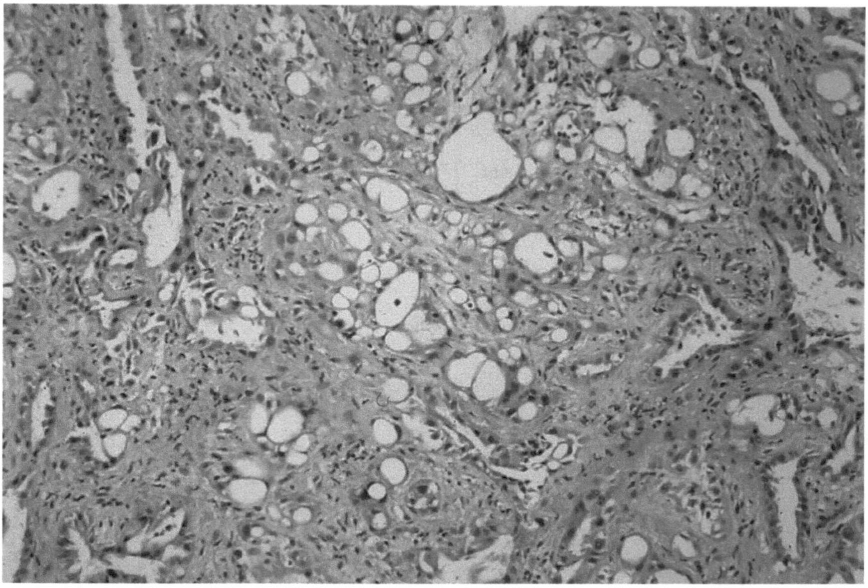

FIGURE 8.5. Macrocystic and microcystic pattern in a mesothelioma.

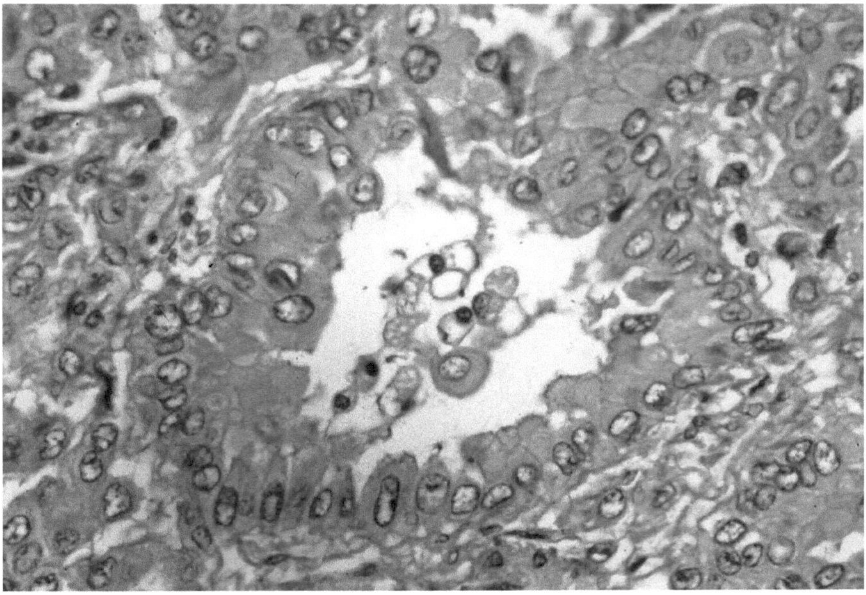

FIGURE 8.6. Mesothelioma containing tubules lined by columnar epithelioid cells.

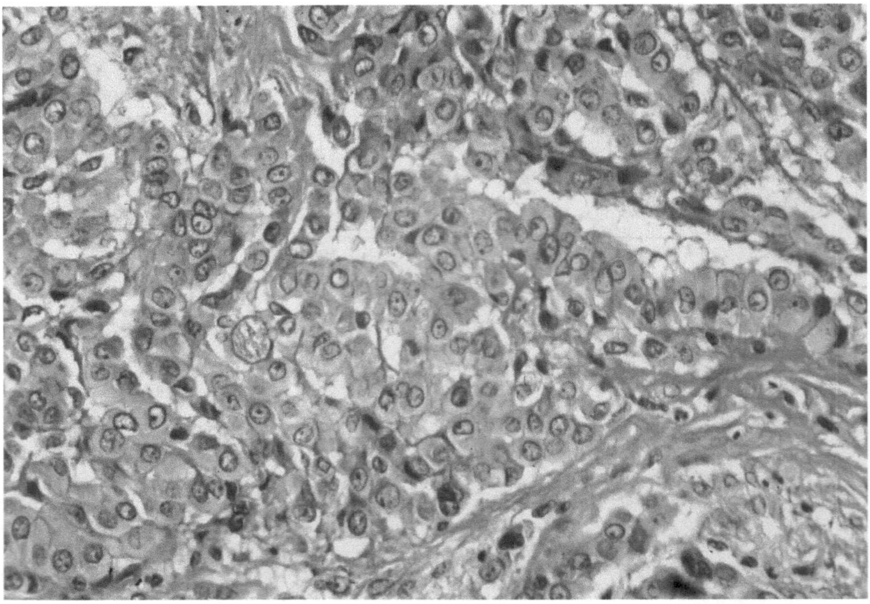

FIGURE 8.7. Mesothelioma with solid sheet of epithelioid cells showing intracytoplasmic vacuoles.

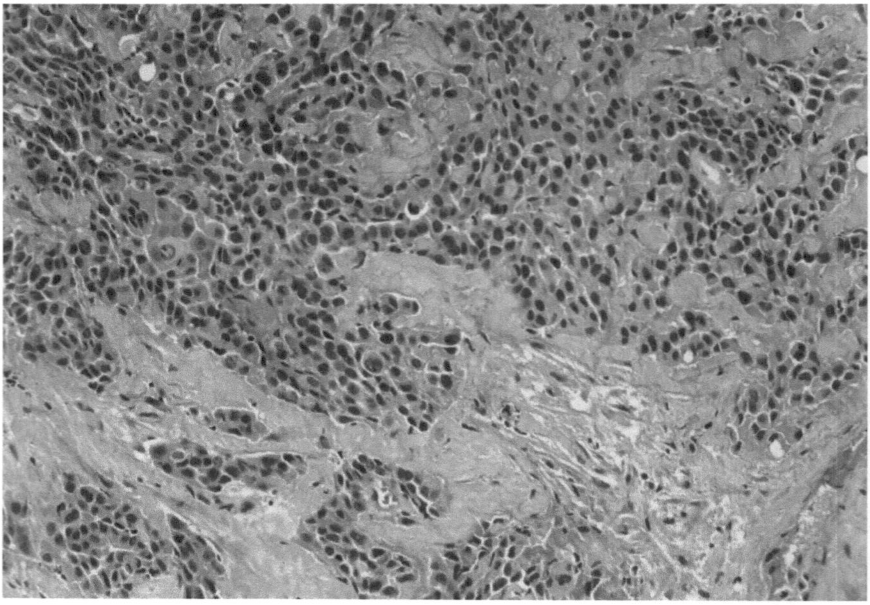

FIGURE 8.8. Low power microscopic appearance showing trabecular pattern in a mesothelioma.

neoplastic cells have the appearance of endometrial decidual cells (endometrial stromal cells transformed by progestational stimulation) (Figure 8.10) [6, 7]. These lesions were initially described in young women not exposed to asbestos but have subsequently been described in older men and in desmoplastic malignant mesothelioma (DMM), but a homogeneous pattern is relatively rare.

Epithelioid mesotheliomas show a wide range of cystic-type changes, including a pattern almost identical to adenoid cystic carcinoma (Figures 8.11 and 8.12). Some mesotheliomas are composed of relatively flattened, innocuous-appearing cells that form microcystic or macrocystic structures. Occasional epithelioid mesotheliomas are composed of cells that contain cytoplasmic vacuoles and have a signet ring morphology but do not stain for neutral mucin (Figures 8.13 and 8.14). Some mesotheliomas produce excessive amounts of secretory products (hyaluronic acid and proteoglycans) and show variable histologic patterns. In some cases, nests of cells lie in lakes of bluish gray, sometimes granular material (Figures 8.15 and 8.16), whereas others show cystic change or have a signet ring morphology (Figure 8.17).

In mesotheliomas that are cystic, it is common to see bluish gray granules in hematoxylin and eosin (H&E)-stained sections in the lumens of cysts or in the individual cytoplasmic lumens (Figure 8.18). When studied ultrastructurally (see below), these granules have the appearance of proteoglycan granules, which have been described within celomic spaces of lower animals.

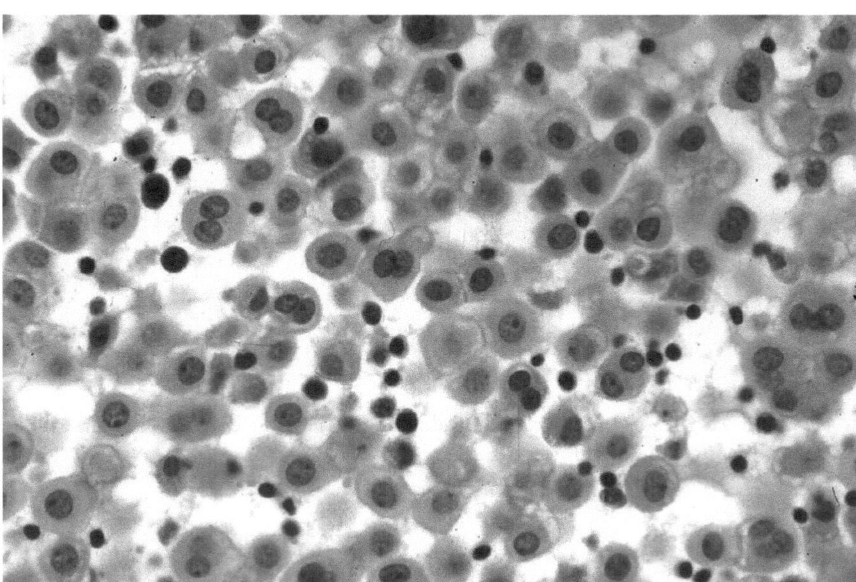

FIGURE 8.9. Noncohesive large "histiocytoid" cells in a mesothelioma.

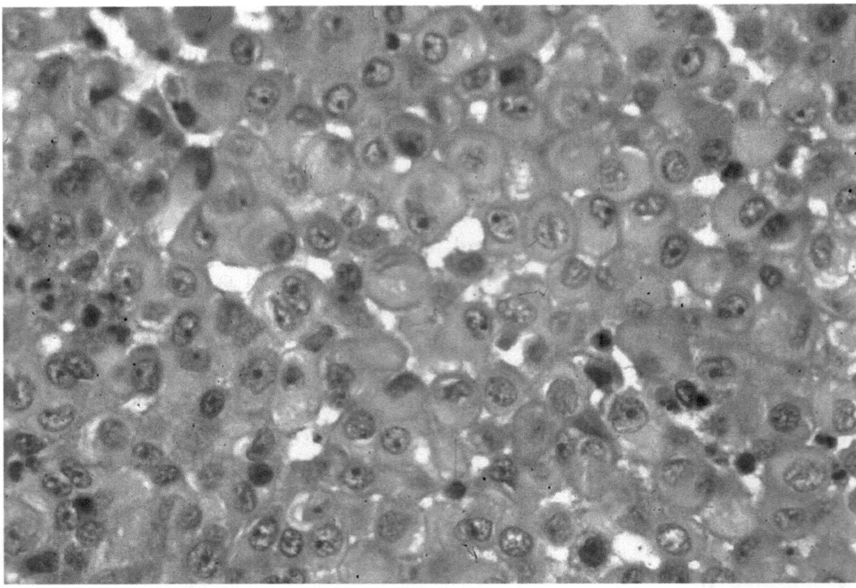

A

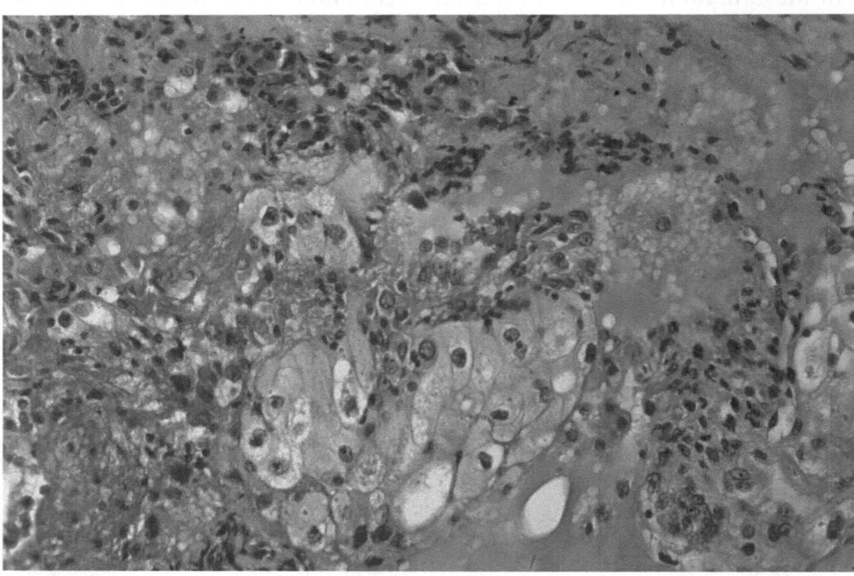

B

FIGURE 8.10. A. Mesothelioma showing deciduoid pattern. B. Mesothelioma with few cells showing the deciduoid pattern.

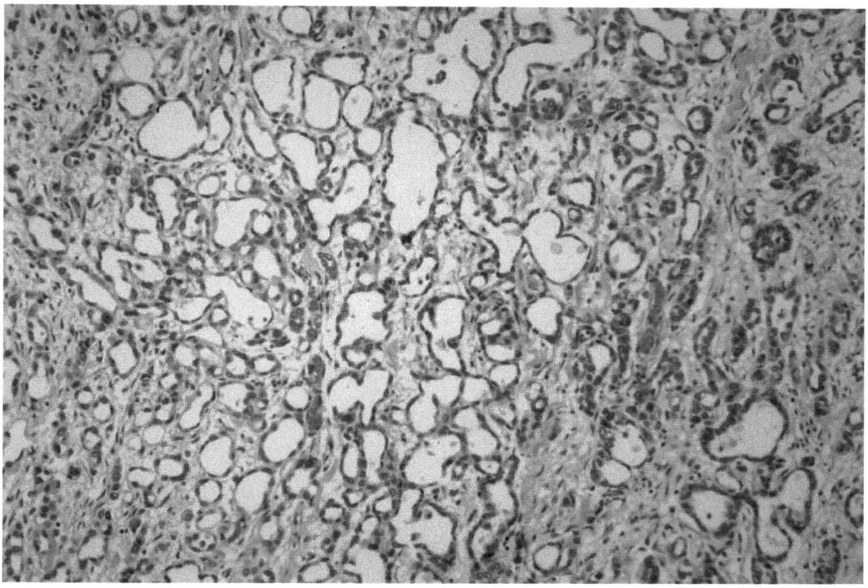

FIGURE 8.11. Microcystic pattern in a mesothelioma.

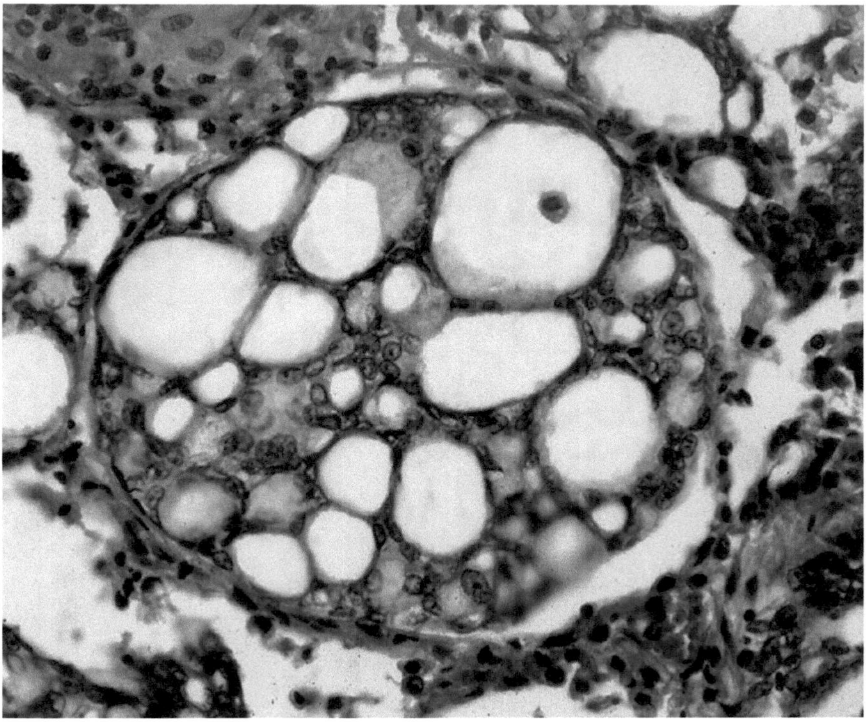

FIGURE 8.12. Adenoid cystic pattern in a mesothelioma.

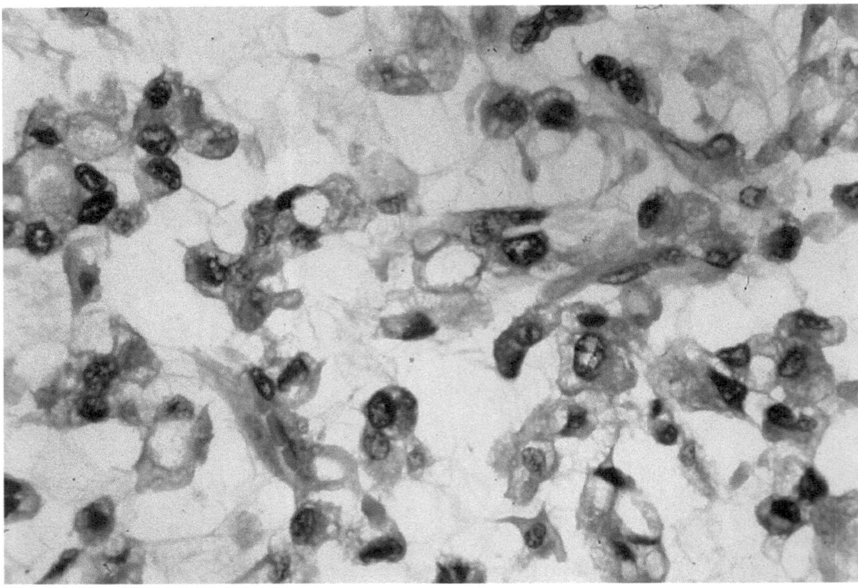

FIGURE 8.13. Mesothelioma showing signet ring cells.

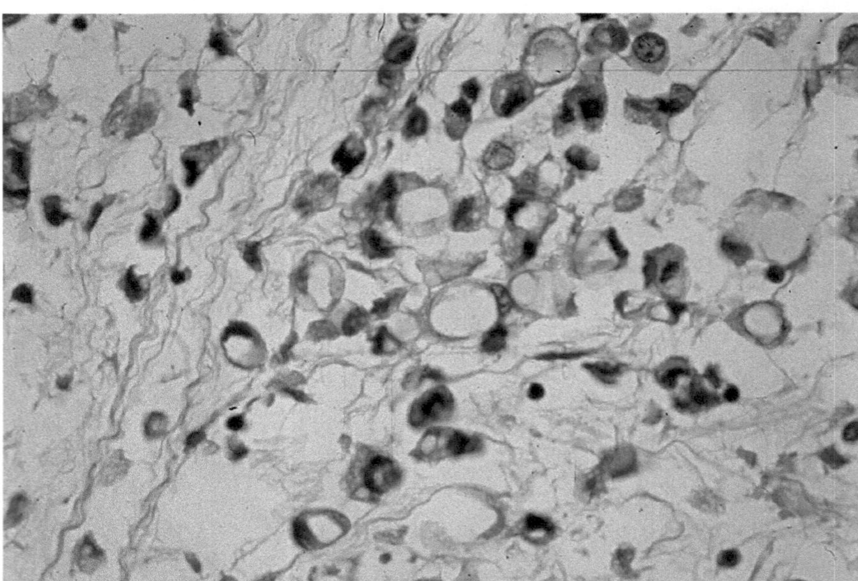

FIGURE 8.14. Mesothelioma showing signet ring cells.

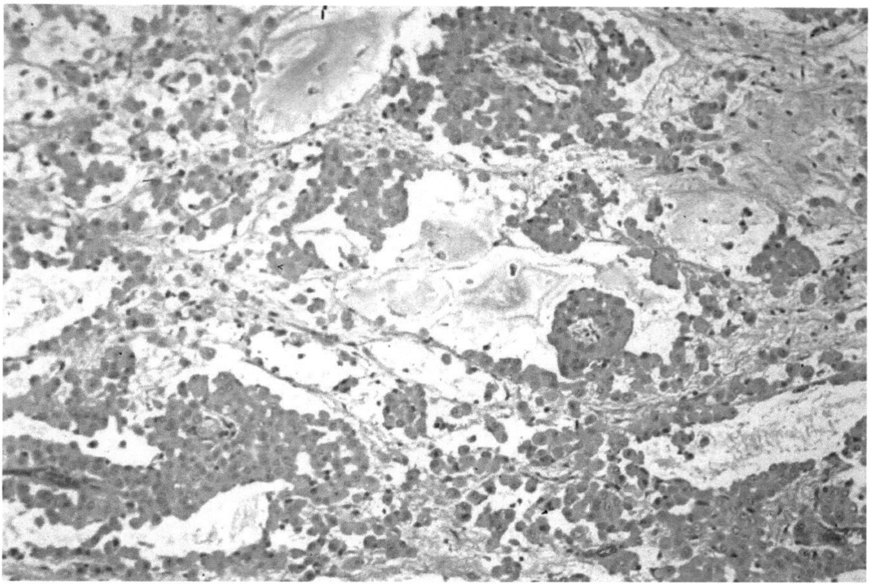

FIGURE 8.15. Mesothelioma showing epithelioid cells lying in lakes of bluish gray material.

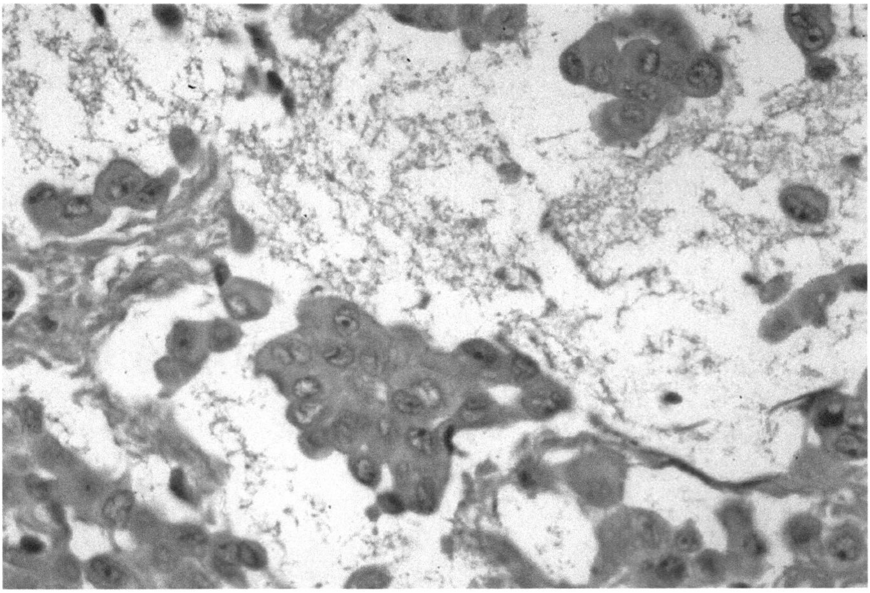

FIGURE 8.16. Epithelioid cells from a mesothelioma floating in pools of mucin.

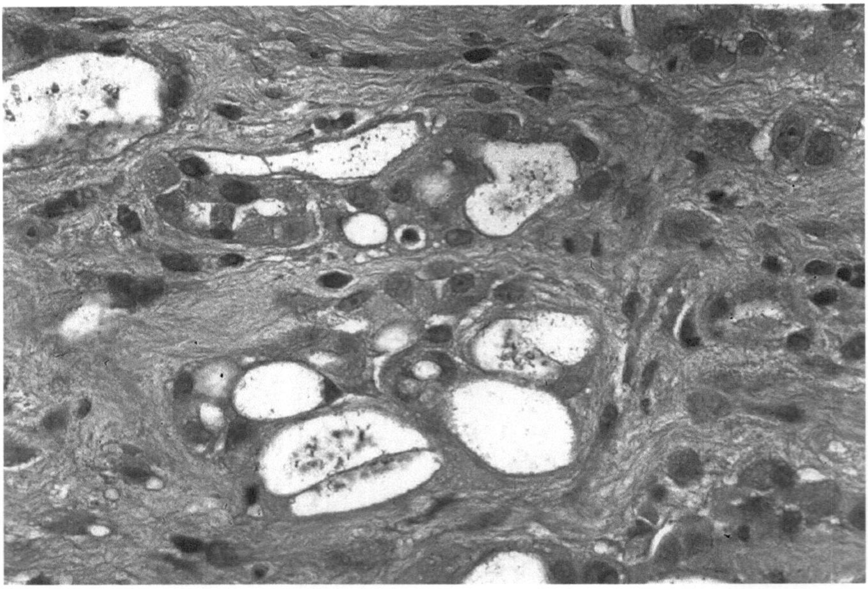

FIGURE 8.17. Mesothelioma containing tubules with fine blue staining in the lumens.

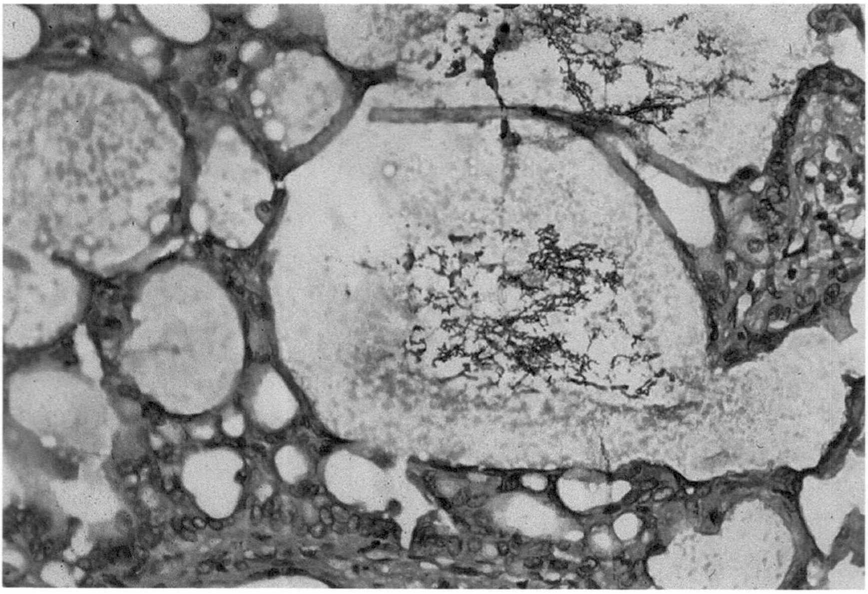

FIGURE 8.18. Mesothelioma showing adenoid cystic pattern with bluish gray material in the lumens.

Some epithelioid mesotheliomas diffusely infiltrate pleura and peritoneal tissue in a single-file arrangement (Figure 8.19) and can be confused with other neoplasms such as metastatic lobular carcinomas of the breast. Few mesotheliomas may have a clear cell appearance mimicking renal cell carcinoma (Figure 8.20). Other mesotheliomas may have a glomeruloid appearance (Figures 8.21 and 8.22), may form a pattern similar to that of chorionic villi seen in the placenta (Figure 8.23), or may grow in a pattern resembling "a pastry roll" (Figures 8.24 and 8.25).

Like neoplasms in other parts of the body, epithelioid mesotheliomas may become poorly differentiated. These mesotheliomas are composed of large anaplastic cells that are round, polygonal, or irregularly shaped (Figures 8.26 through 8.28). These mesotheliomas should be referred to as "poorly differentiated mesotheliomas". They can create a great deal of diagnostic confusion unless it is recognized that they exist (Figure 8.29). Exceptionally, mesotheliomas show a lipidic pattern (Figure 8.29 bis). The poorly differentiated mesotheliomas usually show some immunohistochemical features typical of mesotheliomas. The ultrastructural features of these tumors are usually nonspecific.

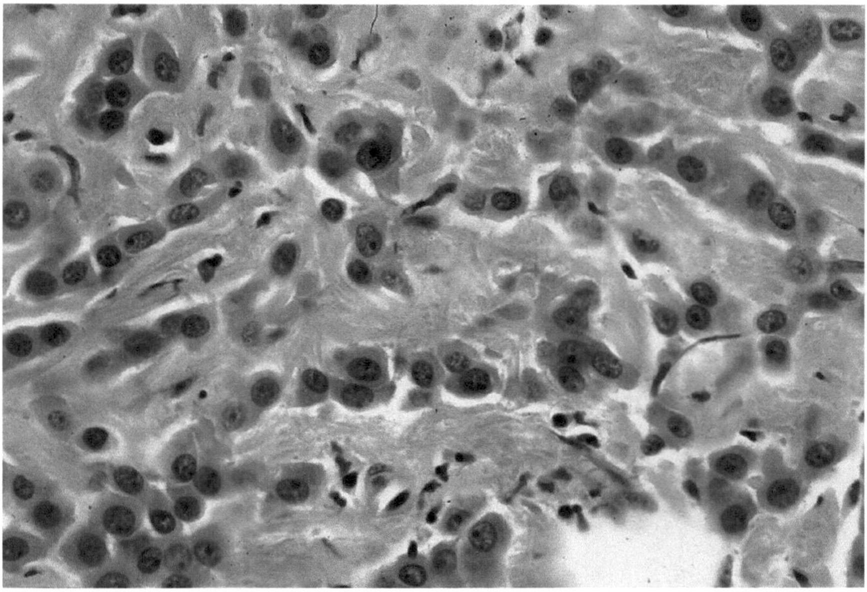

FIGURE 8.19. Mesothelioma showing epithelioid cells arranged in indian file pattern mimicking lobular carcinoma of the breast.

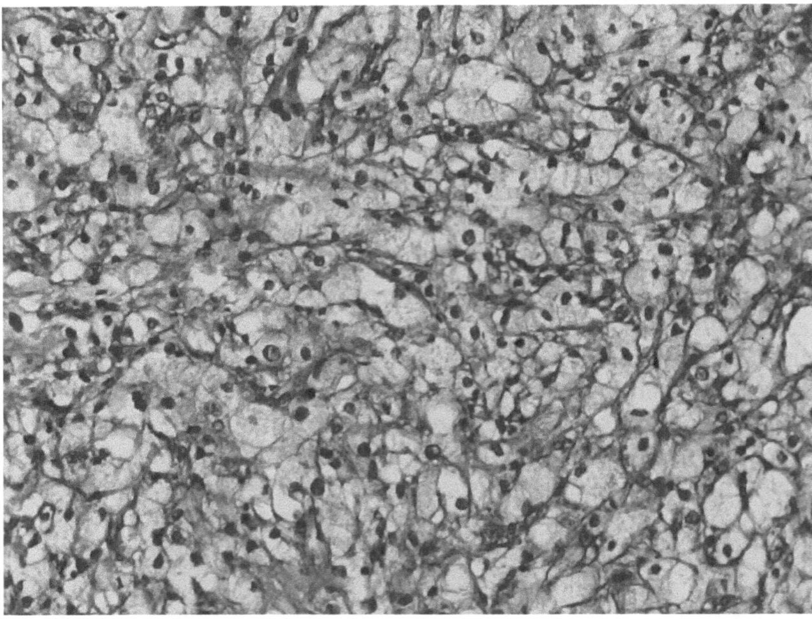

FIGURE 8.20. Mesothelioma with clear cells mimicking renal clear cell carcinoma.

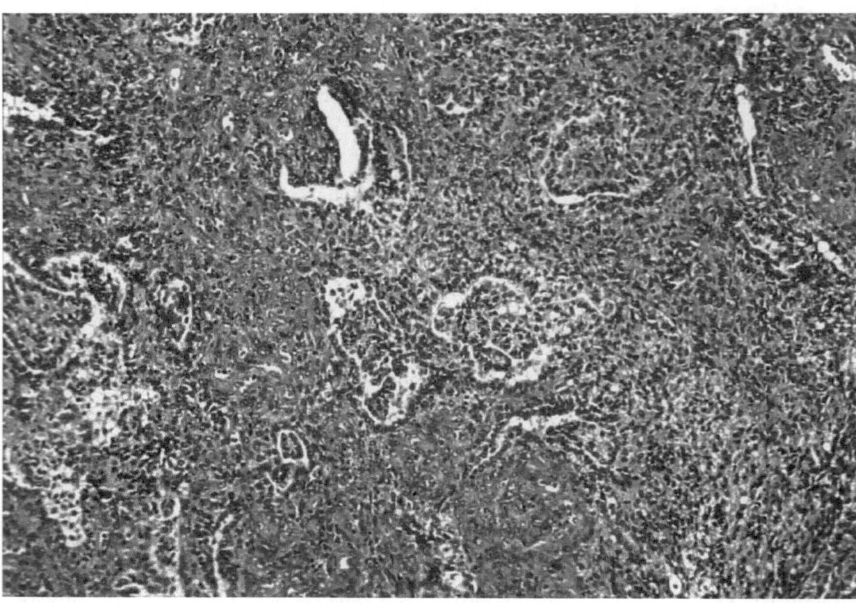

FIGURE 8.21. Mesothelioma with glomeruloid architecture.

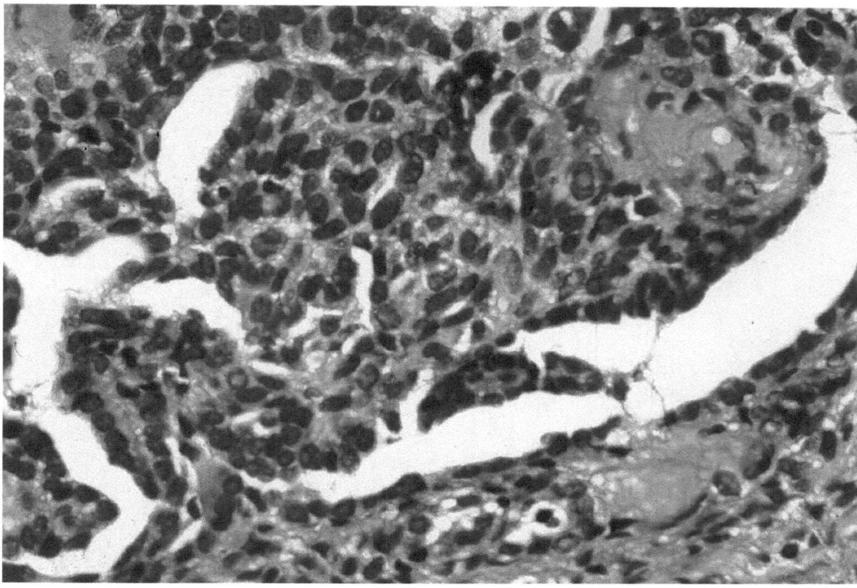

FIGURE 8.22. Glomeruloid architecture at higher power.

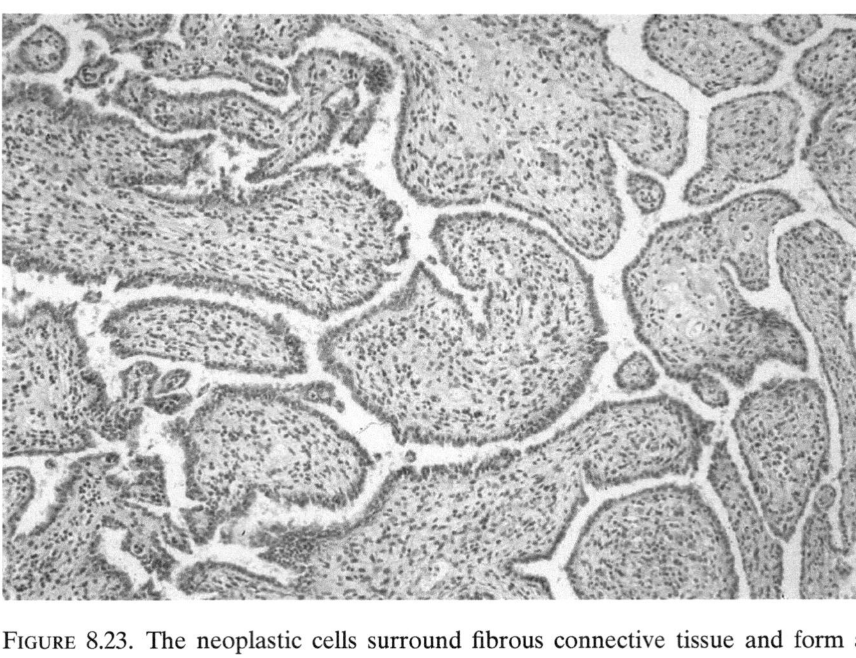

FIGURE 8.23. The neoplastic cells surround fibrous connective tissue and form a pattern mimicking chorionic villi seen in the placenta.

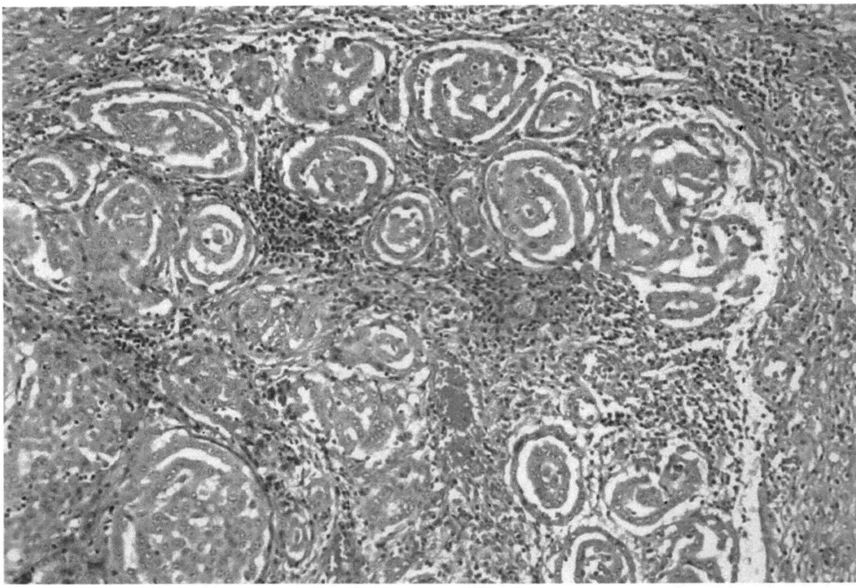

FIGURE 8.24. The neoplastic cells are growing in a pattern resembling a "pastry roll."

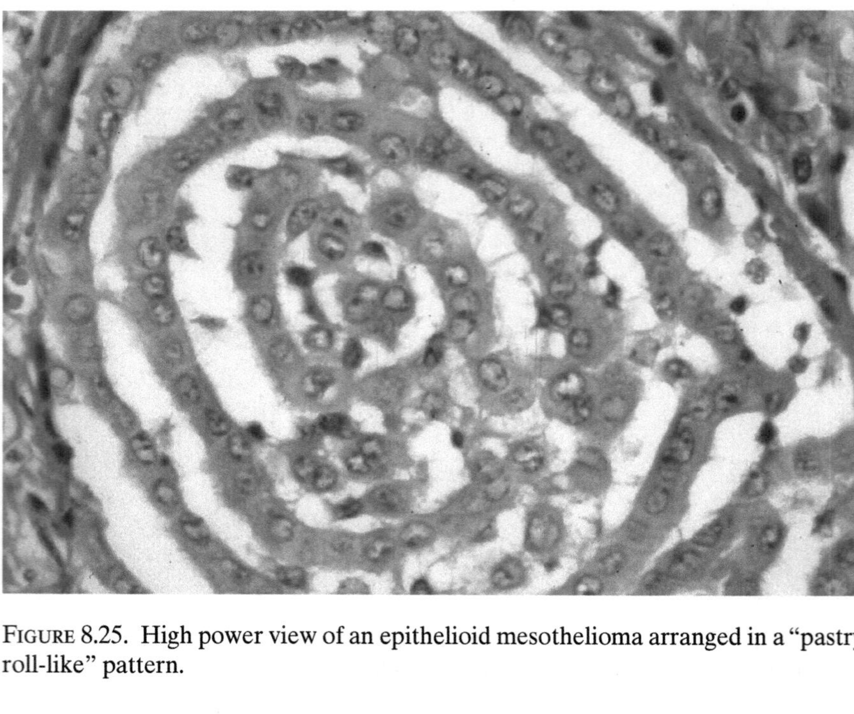

FIGURE 8.25. High power view of an epithelioid mesothelioma arranged in a "pastry roll-like" pattern.

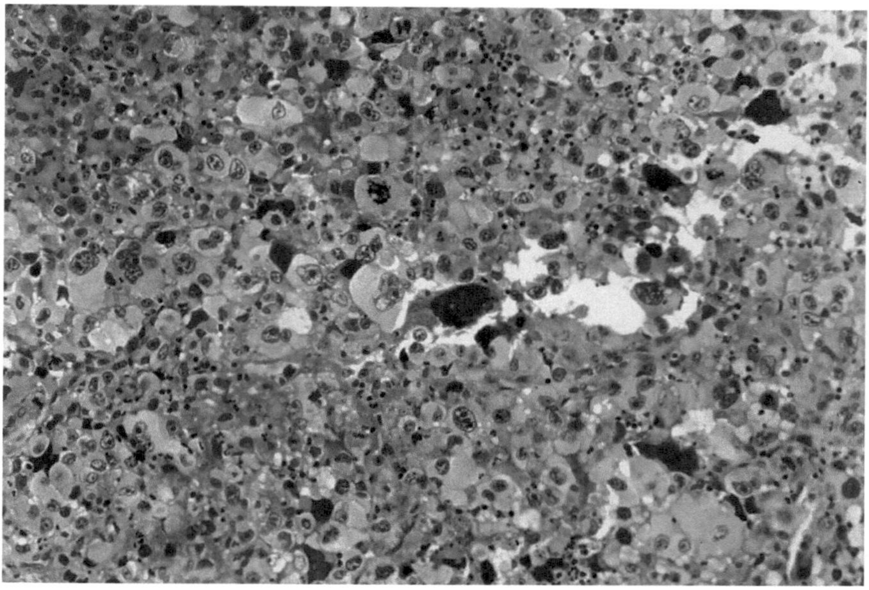

FIGURE 8.26. Low power view of a pleomorphic mesothelioma.

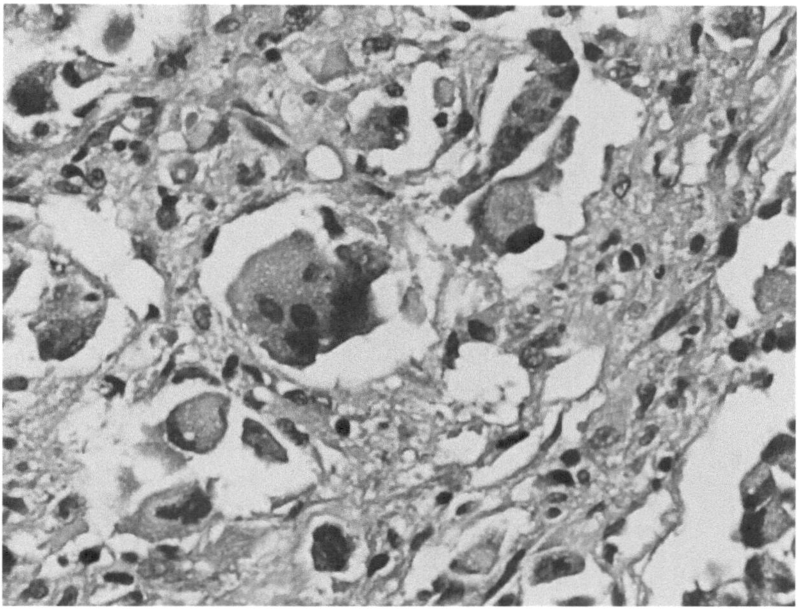

FIGURE 8.27. High power view of a pleomorphic mesothelioma with some tumor giant cells.

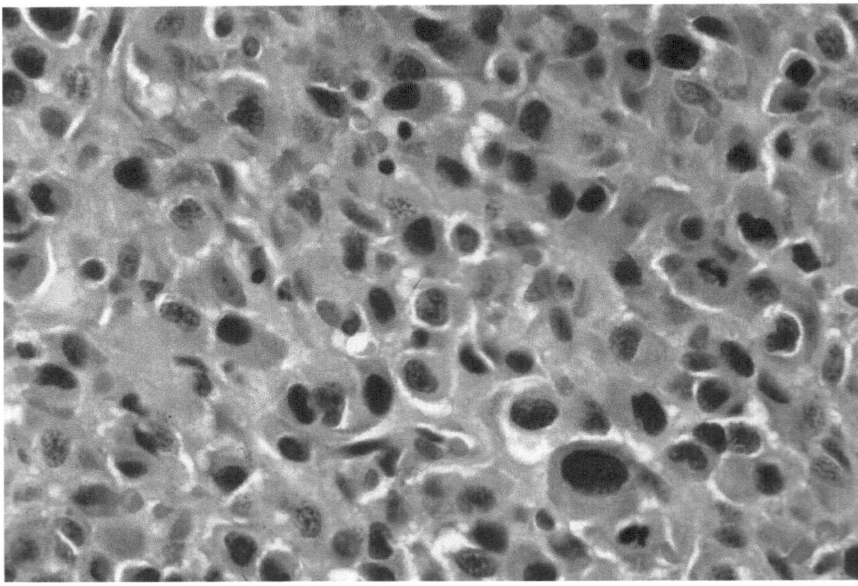

FIGURE 8.28. Pleomorphic mesothelioma showing marked atypia and mitoses.

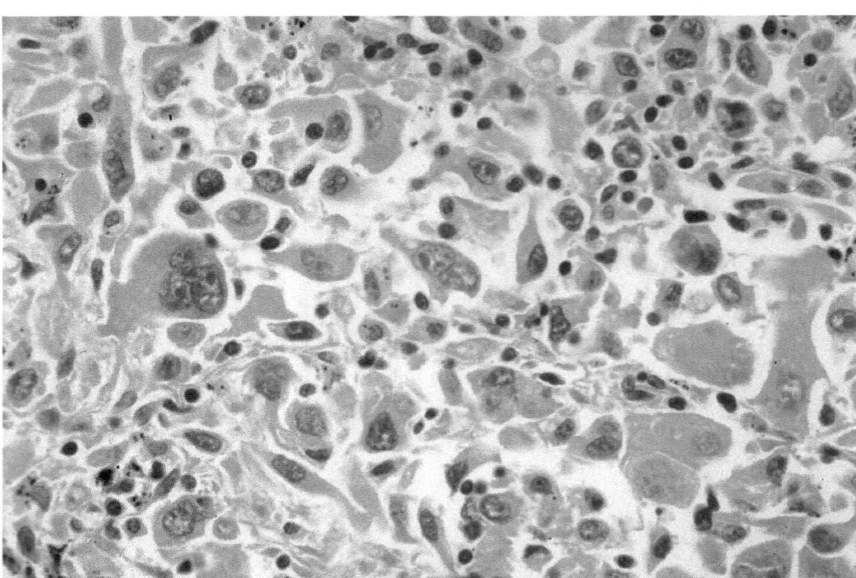

FIGURE 8.29. Reed Sternberg-like cells in a pleomorphic mesothelioma.

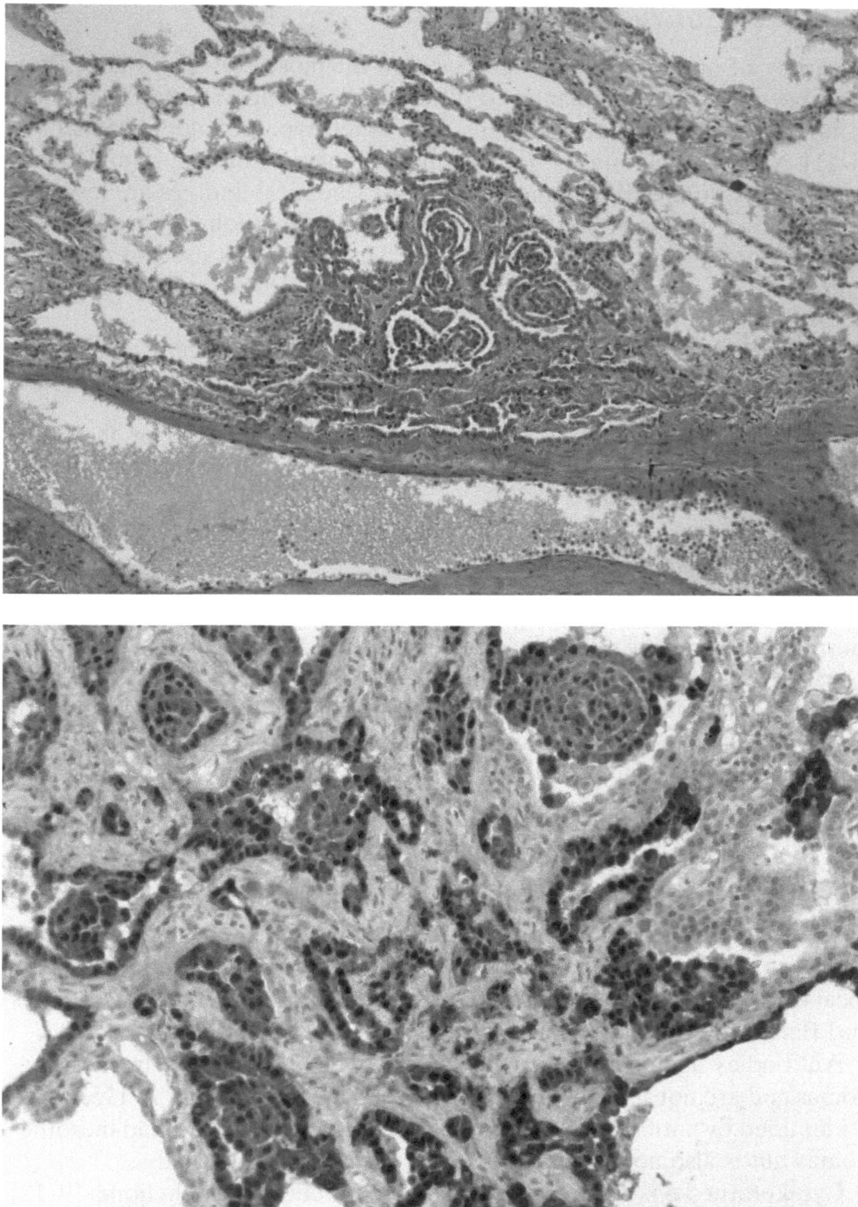

A

B

FIGURE 8.29 bis. A. Epithelioid mesothelioma following interlobular septa. B. Same case: Calretinin immunopositivity.

Immunohistochemical Features

A variety of antibodies have been used to diagnose mesotheliomas. They have been used predominantly to differentiate epithelioid mesotheliomas from pulmonary adenocarcinomas and other types of adenocarcinoma [8–11]. As mesotheliomas or, for that matter, any type of neoplasm become more poorly differentiated, the immunohistochemical findings are less specific. Caution is urged about "overinterpreting" immunohistochemical features in poorly differentiated neoplasms. The antibodies used to diagnose epithelioid mesotheliomas have been divided into three categories.

1. Antibodies that are relatively specific for mesothelial cells and mesotheliomas that, when positive, serve as a positive marker for mesotheliomas
2. Antibodies that show no reaction with mesothelial cells or mesotheliomas and, when positive, serve as a negative marker for mesotheliomas [e.g., estrogen receptors (ERs)
3. Other antibodies that may react with mesothelial cells/mesotheliomas but are relatively nonspecific

Antibodies that are frequently employed in diagnosing (or eliminating) mesotheliomas are listed and characterized in Tables 8.1 and 8.2.

Positive markers include keratin (AE1/AE3, CAM 5.3, KL-1, CK5/6, CK7, CK19) vimentin, calretinin, HBME-1, epithelial membrane antigen/human milk-fat globule protein-2, thrombomodulin, N-cadherin, Wilms' tumor suppressor gene product, and recently mesothelin. Negative markers include carcinoembryonic antigen (CEA), LeuM1 (CD15), B72.3 (TAG-72), BerEP4, MOC-31, BG8, and thyroid transcription factor-1. Some blood group antigens have been observed in mesotheliomas but have also been observed in adenocarcinomas. Thrombomodulin expression has been observed in epithelioid mesotheliomas and in a significant percentage of pulmonary adenocarcinomas. Likewise, epithelioid mesotheliomas show focal expression of CEA, LeuM1 (CD15), and B72.3 in 2% to 10% of cases and BerEP4 in up to 20% of cases and sometimes diffusely.

Antibodies against hyaluronic acid have been evaluated in mesotheliomas and are not specific enough to be used diagnostically. CA-125, which is identified by antibody OC125 or M11 is expressed in epithelioid mesotheliomas but is also not specific enough to be used diagnostically.

Cytokeratin 5/6 is relatively specific for epithelioid mesothelioma [9–12] (Figure 8.30), although it is expressed in squamous cell carcinomas and occasionally other neoplasms such as urothelial carcinomas. Cytokeratin 7 is expressed in nearly 100% of epithelioid mesotheliomas and is expressed in a similar percentage of primary pulmonary adenocarcinomas and a variety of other epithelial neoplasms including breast and esophageal carcinomas. Weak cytokeratin 20 immunostaining is observed in about 10% of epithelioid mesotheliomas. Several reports have suggested that keratin is

Table 8.1. Immunohistochemical markers in epithelioid mesothelioma versus pulmonary adenocarcinoma.

Type of neoplasm	AE1/ AE3	LMWK	HMWK	CK5/6	CK7	Mesothelin	CEA	CD15/ LeuM1	B72.3	BerEP4	TTF-1	Calretinin	HBME-1	EMA	HMFG-2
Epithelioid mesothelioma	+	+	+	+	+	+/–	R	R	R	–/+	N	+/–	+/–[a]	+/–[a]	+/–[a]
Pulmonary adenocarcinoma	+	+	+	–/+	+	R	+	+/–	+/–	+/–	+/–	R	R	+/–[b]	+/–[b]

Reactivity: LMWK, low-molecular-weight keratin; HMWK, high-molecular-weight keratin; CEA, carcinoembryonic antigen; TTF-1, thyroid transcription factor-1; EMA, epithelial membrane antigen; HMFG-2, human milk fat globule protein-2; –/+, variable staining, mostly negative; + almost always diffuse strong positivity; +/– variable staining, mostly positive; R, rare cells positive; N, almost always negative.

[a]Cell membrane distribution.

[b]Cytoplasmic distribution.

Table 8.2. Immunohistochemical spectrum of protein expression in sarcomatoid mesotheliomas.

Vimentin	LMWK	HMWK	Ker 5/6	Calretinin	S-100	smooth cell α-actin	Desmin	CD34	bcl2
+ Always	+>80%	+>80%	+<70%	+~30%	+ Focal <30%	+~30%	+<30%	–	–

See Table 8.1 for abbreviations.

A small percentage of sarcomatoid mesotheliomas are negative for cytokeratins.

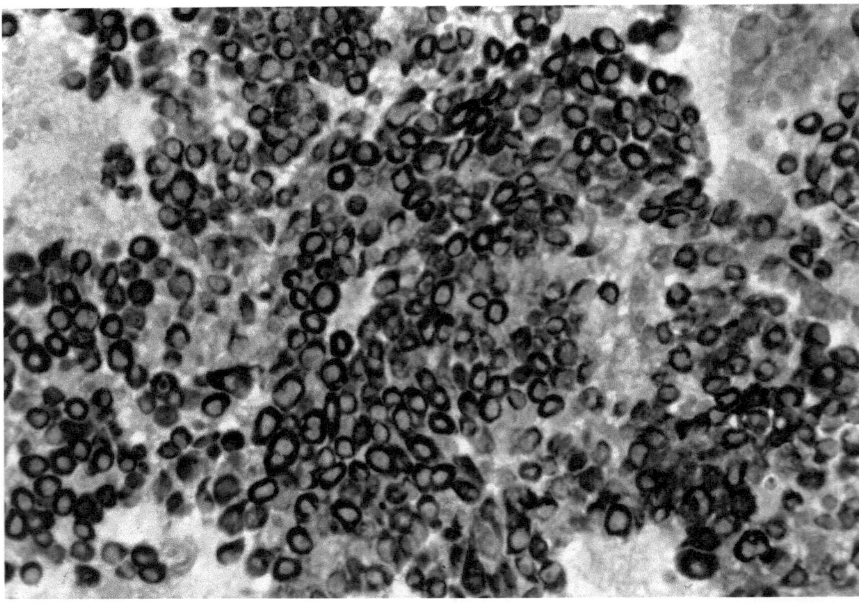

FIGURE 8.30. CK5/6 strong perinuclear immunopositivity in an epithelioid mesothelioma.

more frequently seen in a perinuclear distribution in epithelioid mesotheliomas than in pulmonary adenocarcinomas (Figures 8.31 and 8.32). This is true, but there is too much variability for this finding to be of diagnostic usefulness. The characteristics of various keratins and their expression in epithelioid mesothelioma and pulmonary adenocarcinoma, are shown in Table 8.2.

The intermediate filament vimentin was initially thought to be found only in mesenchyme-derived cells, but it is now recognized that it is expressed in a wide range of tumors not derived from mesenchymal cells. Vimentin has been reported to be more frequently expressed in epithelioid mesotheliomas than in pulmonary adenocarcinomas [13]. This depends to some extent on the differentiation of the tumor; poorly differentiated mesotheliomas demonstrate strong vimentin staining, whereas in well-differentiated mesotheliomas vimentin expression is usually weak or absent. It is well known that mesothelial cells are able to express markers of divergent differentiation. Mesotheliomas may express desmin, and it has been shown that desmin is preferentially expressed in reactive mesothelial cells, rather than in malignant cells [14]. Smooth muscle actin (SMA) and muscle-specific actin (MSA) has also been observed immunohistochemically in both epithelioid and sarcomatoid mesothelioma mesotheliomas, but these markers are not of diagnostic value, as the stromal cells are also expressing SMA and MSA as well as cytokeratin [15–17].

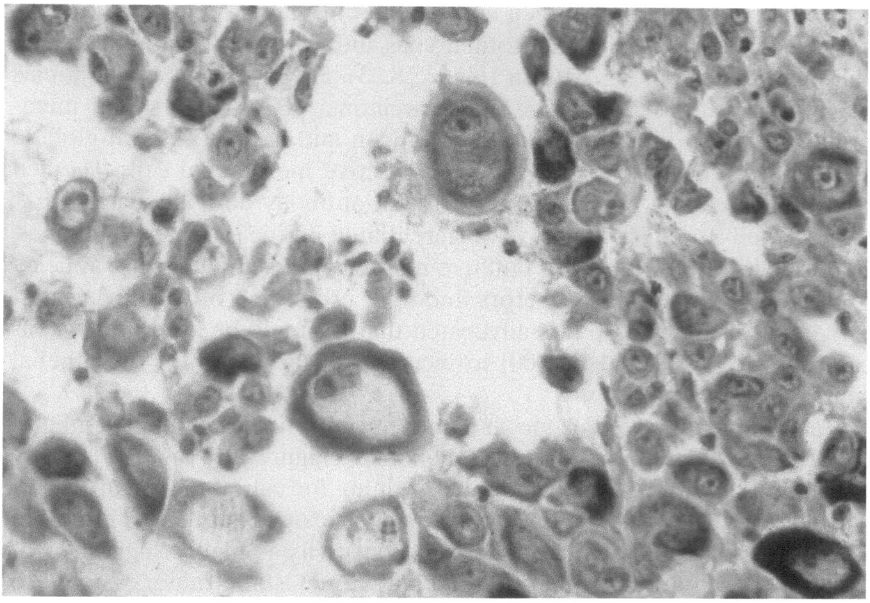

FIGURE 8.31. AE1/AE3 immunopositivity in epithelioid mesothelioma showing the perinuclear and cytoplasmic distribution.

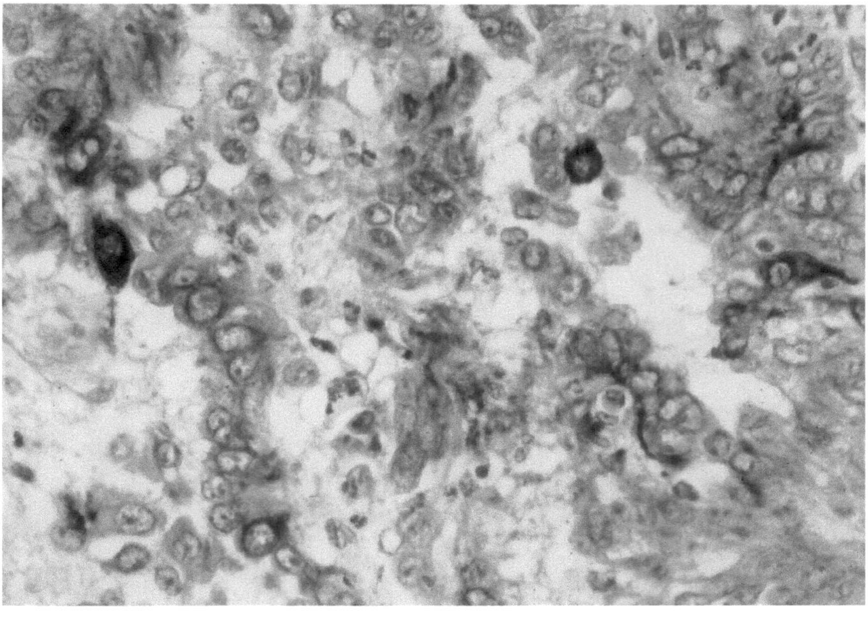

FIGURE 8.32. Strong AE1/AE3 perinuclear positivity of reactive mesothelial cells in comparaison with pericytoplasmic positivity of adenocarcinomatous cells.

Epithelial membrane antigen and human milk fat globule protein-2 are positive in most epithelioid mesotheliomas and show predominantly a thick cell membrane staining pattern (Figure 8.33). However, some carcinomas [e.g., nonmucinous bronchoalveolar carcinoma (BAC)] show cell membrane staining. Epithelial membrane antigen and human milk fat globule protein-2 are usually not expressed in reactive mesothelial cells. The cell membrane staining pattern is seen with an antibody designated HBME-1 in most well- to moderately well-differentiated epithelioid mesotheliomas. Experience with HBME-1, a putative marker of mesothelial cells, appears to vary widely, some investigators finding it useful and others declaring it to be nonspecific [2, 10]. It is advocated that it should be used in low concentration (1:5000 to 1:15,000] to increase its specificity for mesothelial cells.

Heterogeneous cytoplasmic and nuclear calretinin immunostaining is observed in most epithelioid mesotheliomas (Figure 8.34) [18, 19]. Many carcinomas show cytoplasmic immunostaining for calretinin (Figure 8.35), which is a nonspecific reaction and not diagnostic of an epithelioid mesothelioma. We suggest that nuclear staining positivity is highly suggestive of an epithelioid mesothelioma after excluding metastatic tumors known to express calretinin (with nuclear staining). These include urothelial carcinoma that is also CK5/6-positive, granulosa cell tumor but expressing inhibin (mesotheliomas do not), and in rare cases metastatic breast carcinoma that may express calretinin positivity with focal nuclear staining. In

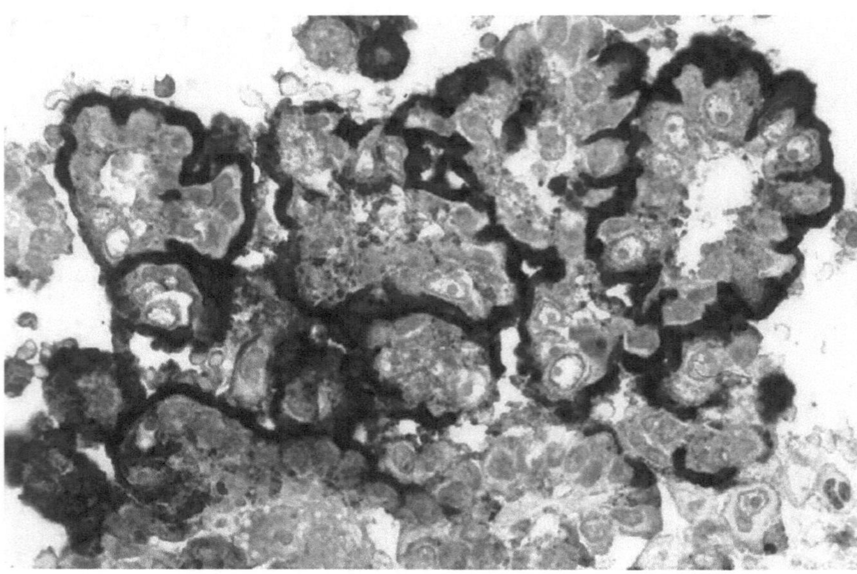

FIGURE 8.33. Epithelial membrane antigen (EMA) membranous staining with thick borders in epithelioid mesothelioma.

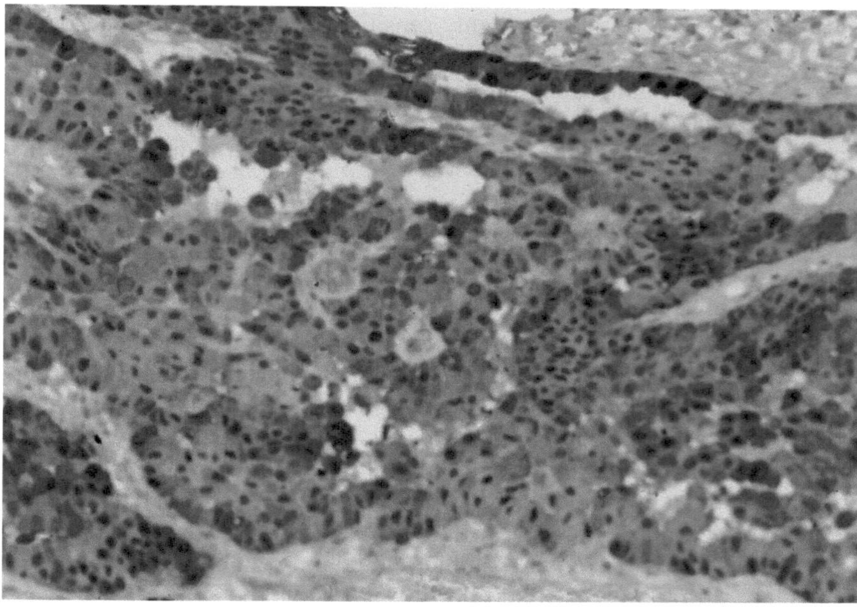

FIGURE 8.34. Neoplastic cells present strong nuclear calretinin staining with a typical fried egg appearance and heterogeneous cytoplasmic staining.

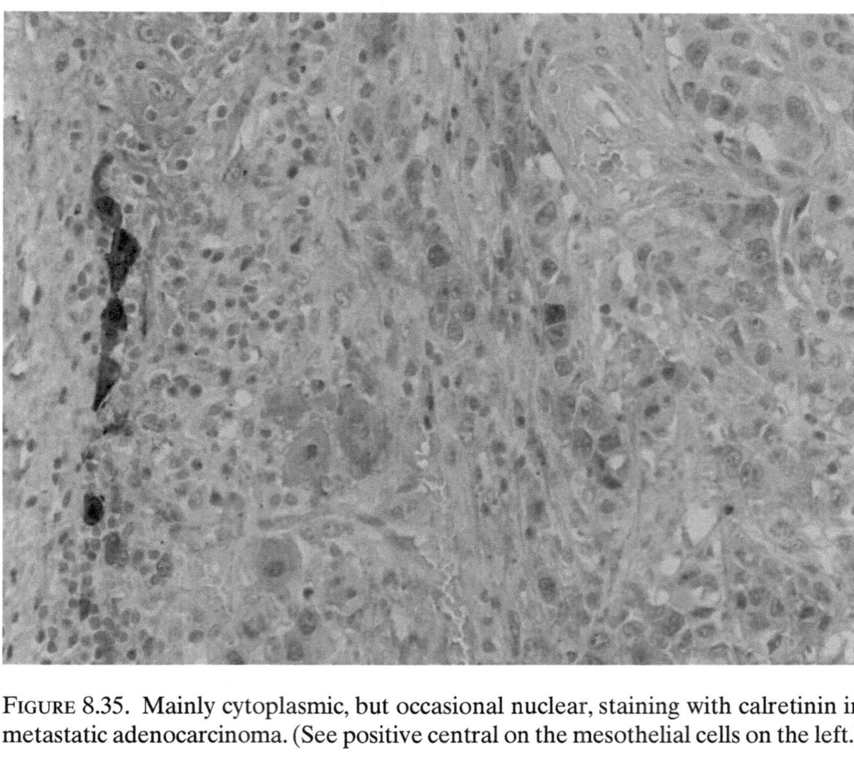

FIGURE 8.35. Mainly cytoplasmic, but occasional nuclear, staining with calretinin in metastatic adenocarcinoma. (See positive central on the mesothelial cells on the left.)

this situation ER negativity is highly sensitive in distinguishing mesothelioma (100% negative) from metastatic breast carcinoma.

Neuroendocrine markers are usually not expressed by benign or malignant mesothelial cells, except for NCAM expression, which occurs in 73% of cases. This is reminiscent of its expression in mesoderm during fetal life [20].

Mesothelin is a cell surface antigen of unknown function with the 5B2 anti-mesothelin antibody, which has only recently become commercially available in formalin-fixed, paraffin-embedded samples. It is strongly expressed in normal mesothelial cells and mesotheliomas, as well as in nonmucinous ovarian carcinomas, pancreatic ductal adenocarcinomas, 40% of lung adenocarcinomas, and in some other malignancies [21]. This marker seems to have more promising diagnostic value as a serum marker of malignancy. Robinson et al. demonstrated that 84% of 44 patients with mesothelioma had elevated concentrations of soluble related mesothelin protein compared with 2% of 160 patients with other cancers or other inflammatory lung or pleural diseases, and with none of 28 controls who had not been exposed to asbestos. Moreover, soluble related mesothelin protein appears to correlate with tumor size and tumor progression [22, 23].

With respect to the immunohistochemical markers of epithelioid mesotheliomas, there is no antibody that is 100% specific and 100% sensitive. The specificities and sensitivities of various antibodies used for diagnosing mesothelioma have been evaluated, and different results have been found by different investigators [24, 25]. For this reason, most tumors suspected to be epithelioid mesotheliomas are evaluated with a panel of antibodies looking for the positive and negative reactions. Preferred markers depend on the experience of the laboratory but the International Mesothelioma Panel recommends the use of at least two positive and two negative mesothelioma markers and a broad spectrum cytokeratin as an initial panel. If these results are not conclusive, additional mesothelial, epithelial, vascular, or melanoma markers may be necessary.

Ultrastructural Features

The ultrastructural features of epithelioid mesotheliomas depend on the histologic/cytologic appearance of the mesothelioma evaluated. Electron microscopy can be diagnostic for epithelioid mesotheliomas, particularly when immunohistochemical staining results are discordant. The ultrastructural features have been extensively described [26–30]. In general, the most specific features of well-differentiated and moderately—well-differentiated epithelioid mesotheliomas are long, thin, sinuous microvilli that arise from the cell surface (Figures 8.36 and 8.37). Comparisons have been made between the length/width ratios of the microvilli of epithelioid mesotheliomas and various adenocarcinomas. In general, this exercise is not worth the time spent to do it in that it is difficult to determine length/width ratios of epithelioid mesotheliomas because the microvilli are not straight. In

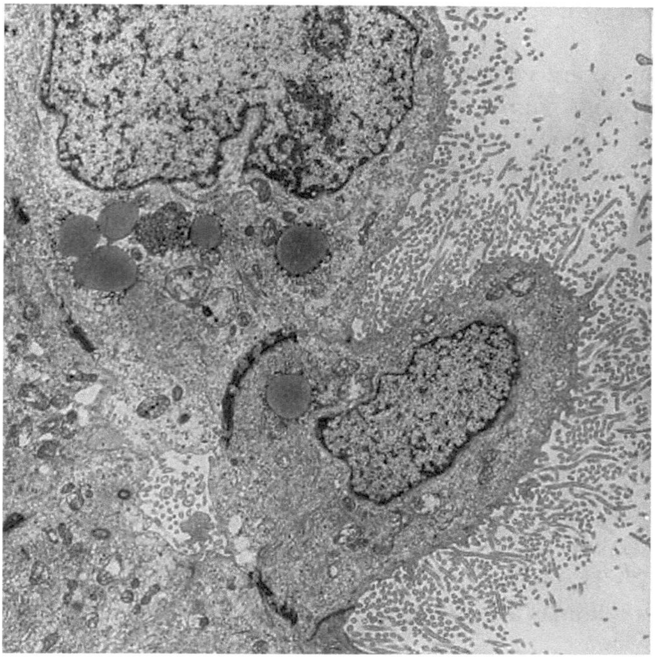

FIGURE 8.36. Ultrastructurally, epithelioid mesotheliomas are composed of neoplastic cells that have long, thin, sinuous microvilli.

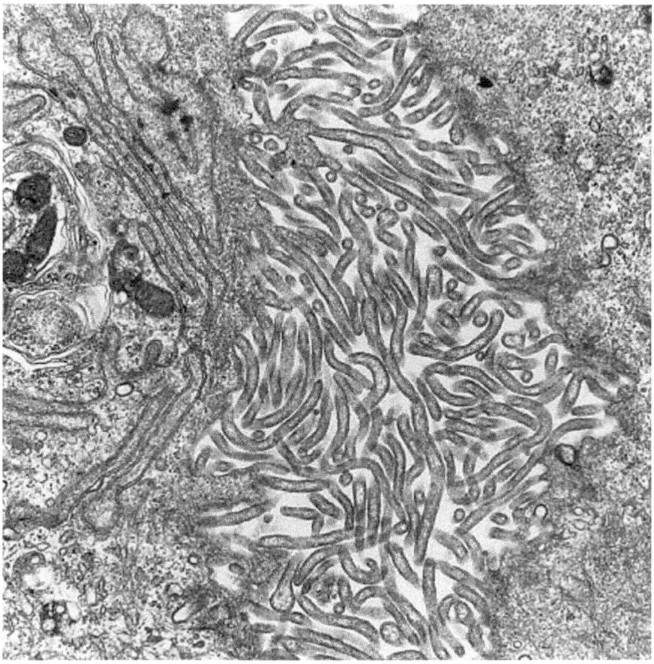

FIGURE 8.37. Epithelioid mesothelioma. The long, thin microvilli are not covered by glycocalyx like that seen in adenocarcinomas.

addition, there are various ultrastructural features that help differentiate epithelioid mesotheliomas from pulmonary and other adenocarcinomas. The surface of the microvilli of epithelioid mesotheliomas is smooth, with the exception that in epithelioid mesotheliomas that produce excess amounts of hyaluronic acid/proteoglycans there can be medium electron-dense material on the surface of the microvilli (Figure 8.38). Sometimes the microvilli appear to be embedded in this material (Figure 8.39). In contrast, most pulmonary adenocarcinomas and many other adenocarcinomas are associated with glycocalyceal bodies (Figure 8.40) and have a fuzzy glycocalyx covering on their surfaces. In addition, the microvilli of most pulmonary and other adenocarcinomas are straight (Figure 8.41). Rare pulmonary adenocarcinomas have long, thin, relatively sinuous microvilli, but in our experience these are always covered by a fuzzy glycocalyx, which is the differentiating feature used to distinguish pulmonary adenocarcinoma from epithelioid mesothelioma [31]. Many pulmonary adenocarcinomas show rootlets in the apical cytoplasm in association with their microvilli (Figure 8.42). These are not seen in epithelioid mesotheliomas. Most epithelioid mesotheliomas are connected to each other by junctional complexes

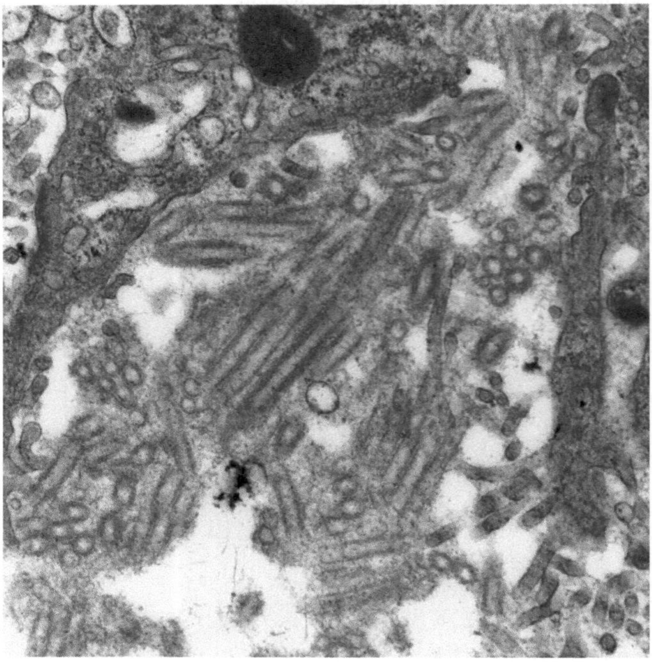

FIGURE 8.38. In epithelioid mesotheliomas producing excess amounts of hyaluronic acid proteoglycans, the microvilli are occasionally covered by a medium electron-dense material.

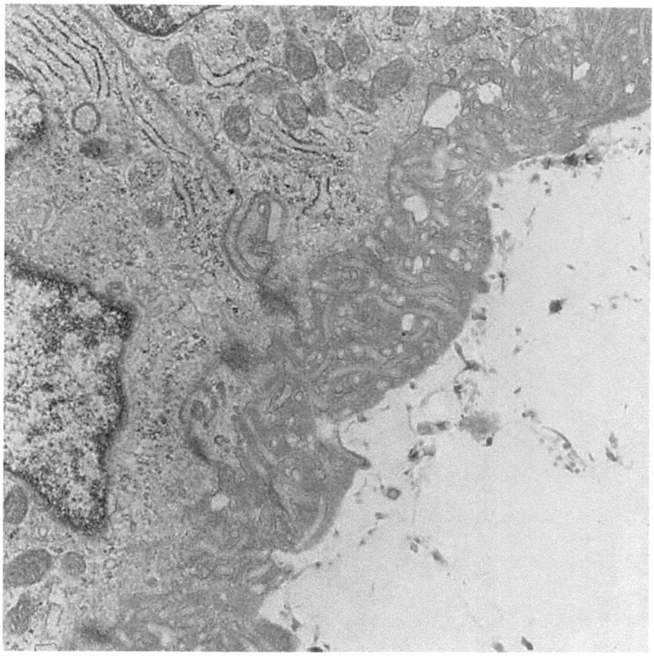

FIGURE 8.39. In mesotheliomas producing excess amounts of hyaluronic acid or proteoglycan, the microvilli can be embedded in this material.

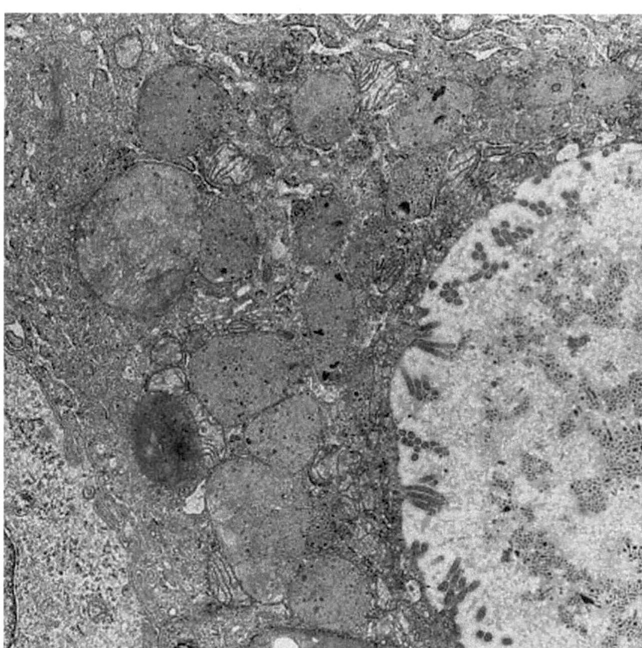

FIGURE 8.40. In contrast to epithelioid mesotheliomas, the microvilli are usually associated with glycocalyceal bodies in adenocarcinomas.

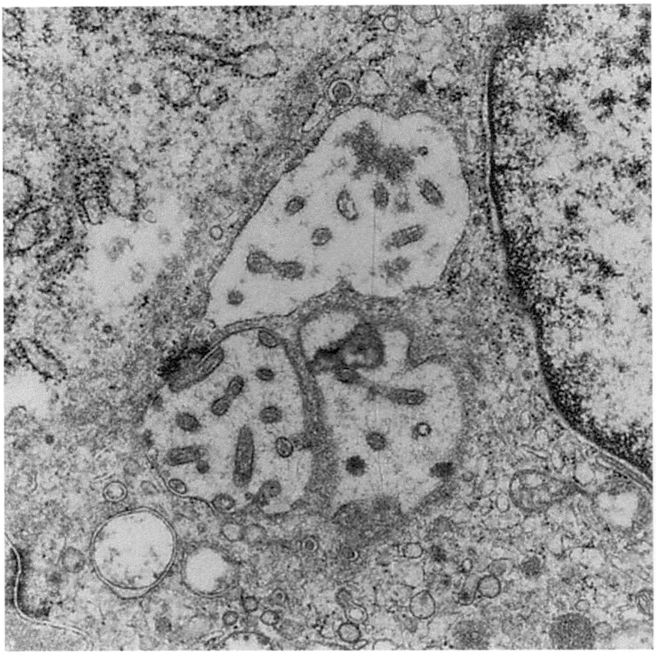

FIGURE 8.41. Most pulmonary adenocarcinomas and other nonpulmonary adenocarcinomas have relatively straight, short microvilli.

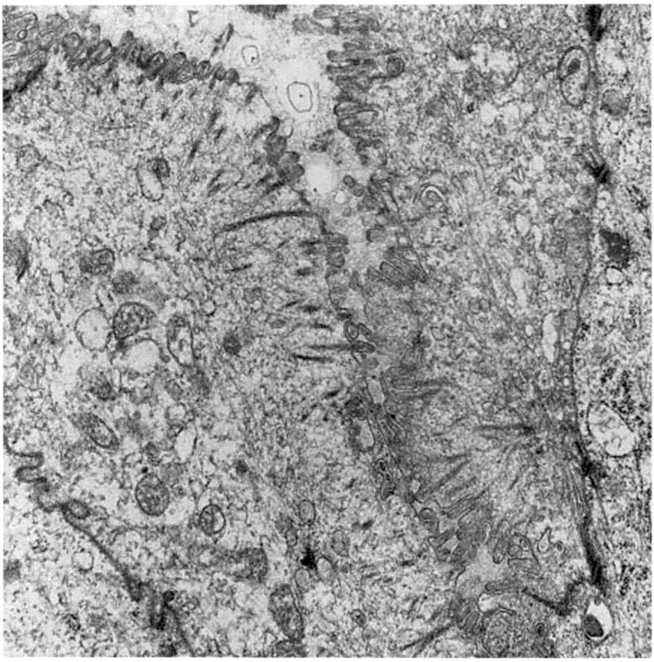

FIGURE 8.42. Pulmonary adenocarcinoma, showing rootlets in the apical cytoplasm in association with their microvilli.

and large desmosomes (Figure 8.43), more frequently seen than in pulmonary or other adenocarcinomas. The microvilli of epithelioid mesothelioma frequently project into adjacent extracellular collagen, a finding referred to as the microvillous-matrix interaction (Figure 8.44).

The distribution of intermediate filaments, specifically keratin filaments, has been evaluated in epithelioid mesotheliomas. In general, epithelioid mesotheliomas more frequently show intermediate keratin filaments in a perinuclear distribution than is seen in adenocarcinomas. This is not an absolute finding, however, as some adenocarcinomas have tonofilaments in a perinuclear distribution and some epithelioid mesotheliomas have relatively diffuse intermediate keratin filaments throughout their cytoplasm. Adenocarcinomas of the lung and other organs may produce packaged mucin in the form of cytoplasmic granules. These granules in pulmonary adenocarcinomas exhibit a wide range of ultrastructural appearances, and they must be appreciated. In contrast, the secretory products of epithelioid mesotheliomas (hyaluronic acid/proteoglycans) are not packaged in the cell but are secreted onto the surface of mesothelial cells, with enzymes in the cell membrane being important in the final production of these substances.

In the tumors that produce large amounts of proteoglycans, proteoglycan granules are seen on the surface of the neoplastic cells and in lumens

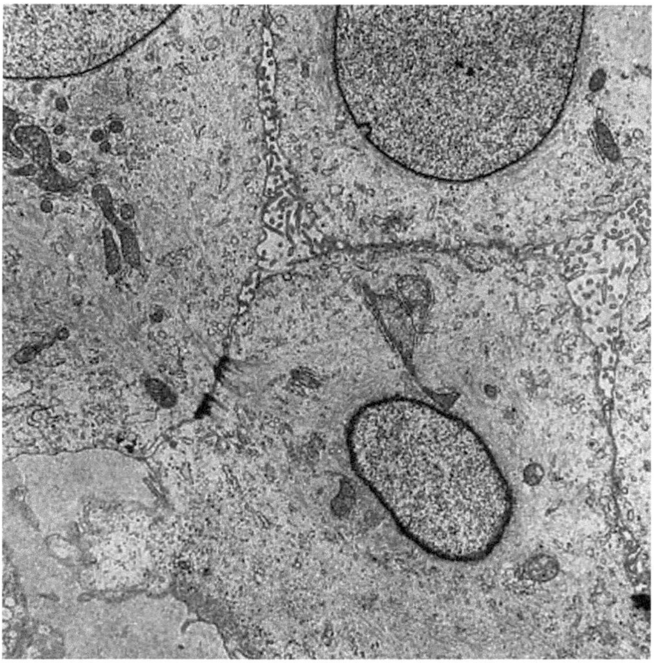

FIGURE 8.43. Epithelioid mesothelial cells connected to each other by junctional complexes and large desmosomes.

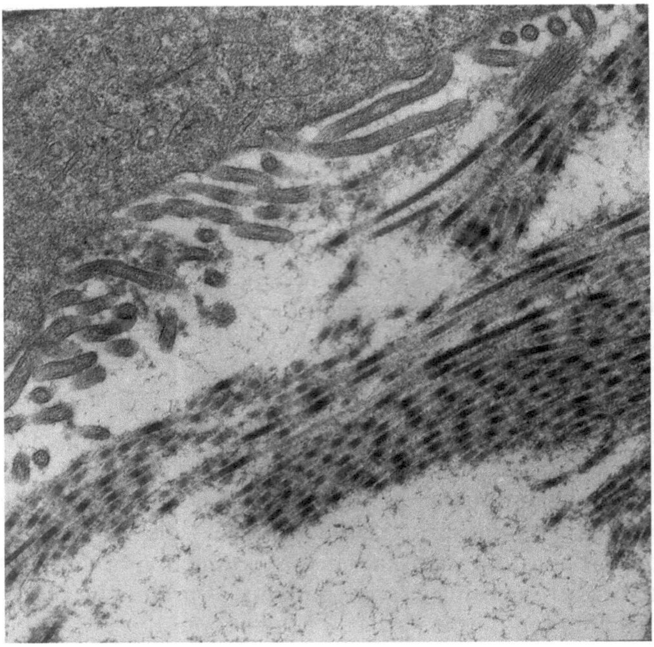

FIGURE 8.44. Microvilli in an epithelioid mesothelioma projecting into adjacent extracellular collagen.

formed by several tumor cells or in intracellular neolumens formed in individual malignant cells. These correlate histologically with the bluish gray granules seen in glandular lumens. These proteoglycan granules are not specific for neoplastic epithelioid mesotheliomas, although they are seen much more commonly in neoplastic mesothelial cells than in normal or reactive mesothelial cells and in other carcinomas.

Tubular crystalloid structures are frequent in mucin-positive epithelioid mesotheliomas [32, 33]. They resemble hollow chrysotile fibers in cross section and are rod-like in longitudinal section. We have seen them only in epithelioid mesotheliomas that are mucin-positive and not in other neoplasms. These crystalloid structures are most likely either abnormal proteoglycans or hyaluronic acid. Rarely, these structures are in the cytoplasm of epithelioid mesotheliomas.

The Gaucher-like cells seen in rare epithelioid mesotheliomas have a characteristic ultrastructural appearance with laminated layers of crystalloid material in the cisterna of the rough endoplasmic reticulum (Figure 8.45).

The deciduoid mesotheliomas have a variety of cellular organelles in their cytoplasm, including intermediate filaments, endoplasmic reticulum, and mitochondria, among others. The microvilli of many of the deciduoid

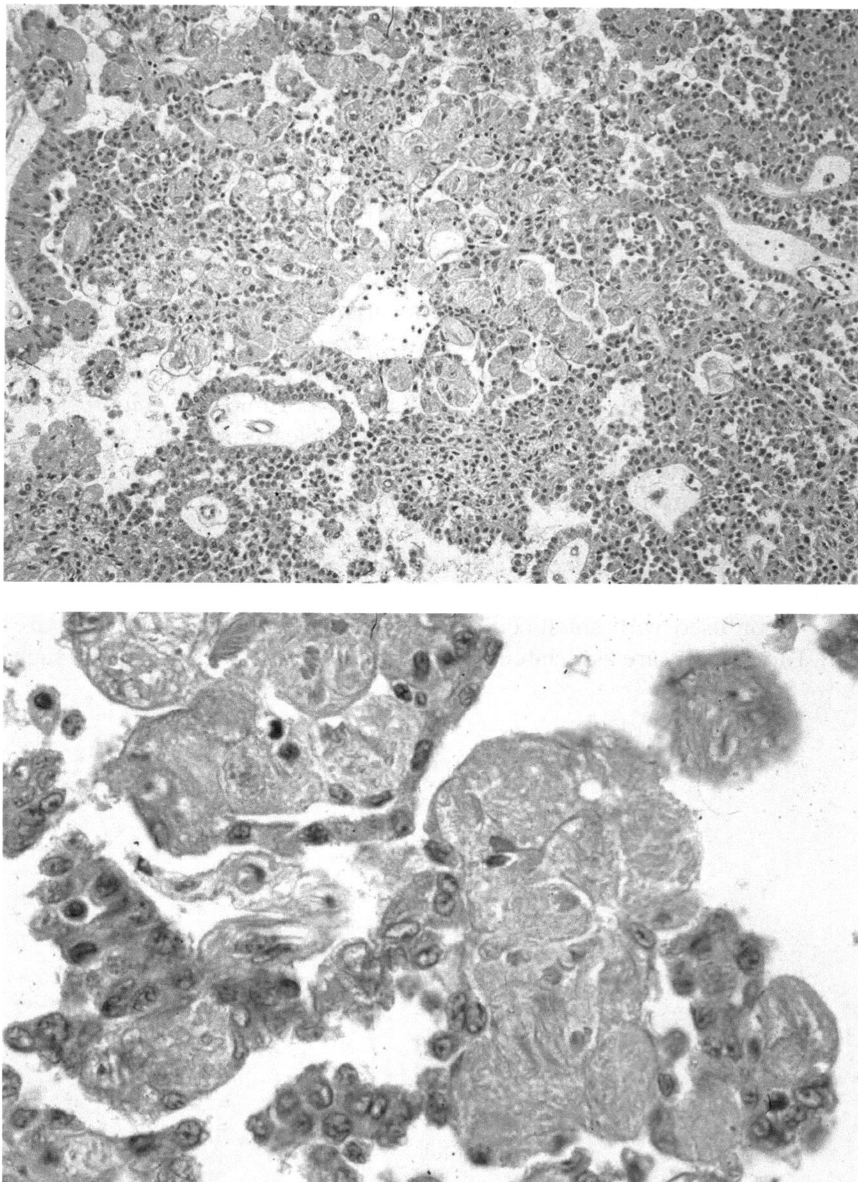

A

B

FIGURE 8.45. A. Gaucher-like cells seen in rare epithelioid mesotheliomas have a characteristic ultrastructural appearance with laminated layers of crystalloid material in the cisterna of the rough endoplasmic reticulum. B. Same case: high power view.

mesotheliomas are shorter than one sees in other epithelioid mesotheliomas. Occasional deciduoid mesotheliomas produce proteoglycan granules.

Rare Forms (Variants) of Epithelioid Mesothelioma

Epithelioid mesotheliomas that produce proteoglycans or hyaluronic acid (or both) can stain positively with mucin stains, usually mucicarmine, and rarely PAS-diastase [Figures 8.46 and 8.47) [32, 33]. These mesotheliomas may be confused with pulmonary adenocarcinomas. In the case of mucicarmine, the material present in the cystic structures or in an extracellular location is usually eradicated if the tissue is pretreated with hyaluronidase, which suggests that the material stained was hyaluronic acid (Figures 8.48 and 8.49). In epithelioid mesotheliomas with mucicarmine or PAS-diastase intracellular droplet-like staining, it is usually not eradicated by pretreatment with hyaluronic acid. In mesotheliomas that have this pattern, the material in the lumens of the neoplastic cells usually has a crystalloid morphology when evaluated ultrastructurally and is described above.

Some mesotheliomas are composed almost entirely of small cells and may be confused with small-cell neuroendocrine neoplasms [34] (Figure 8.50). They usually are associated with other patterns of mesothelioma, such

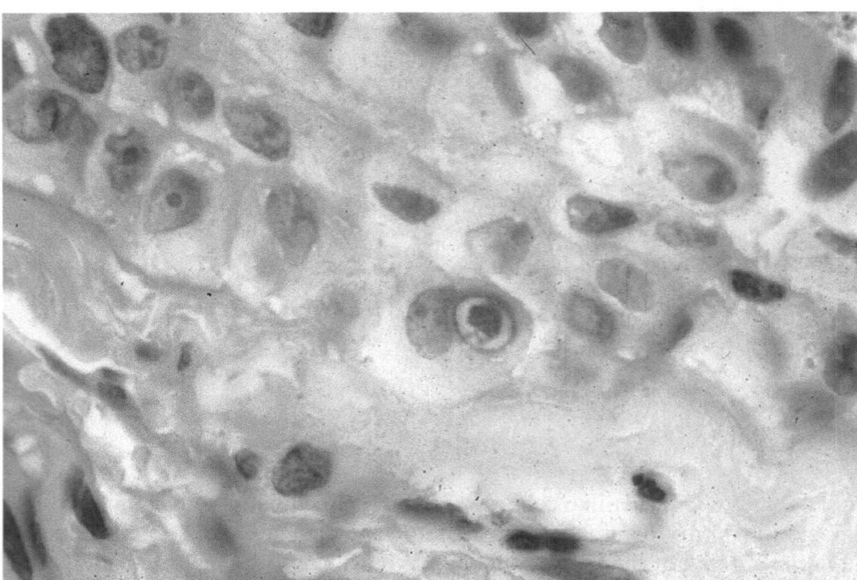

FIGURE 8.46. Epithelioid mesotheliomas that produce proteoglycans, hyaluronic acid, or both can stain positively with mucin stains, usually mucicarmine, and rarely periodic acid-Schiff (PAS) diastase.

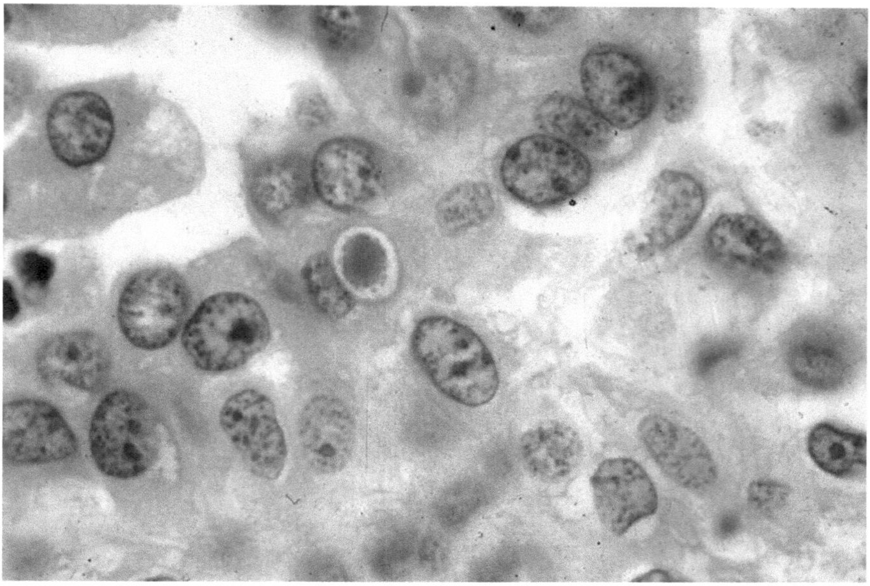

FIGURE 8.47. Same case as in Figure 8.46 but with mucicarmine stains.

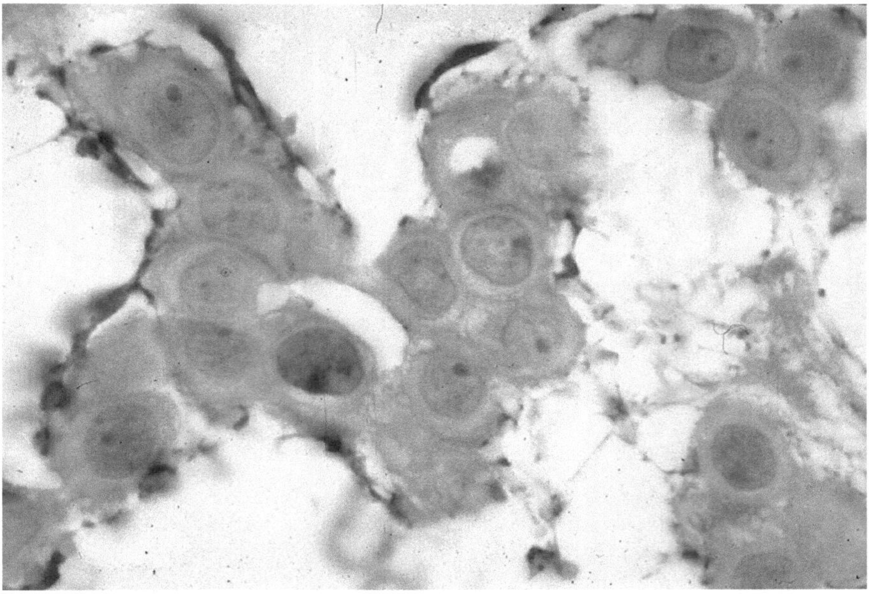

FIGURE 8.48. Epithelioid mesotheliomas that produce proteoglycans, hyaluronic acid, or both stain positively with mucin stains, such as mucicarmine.

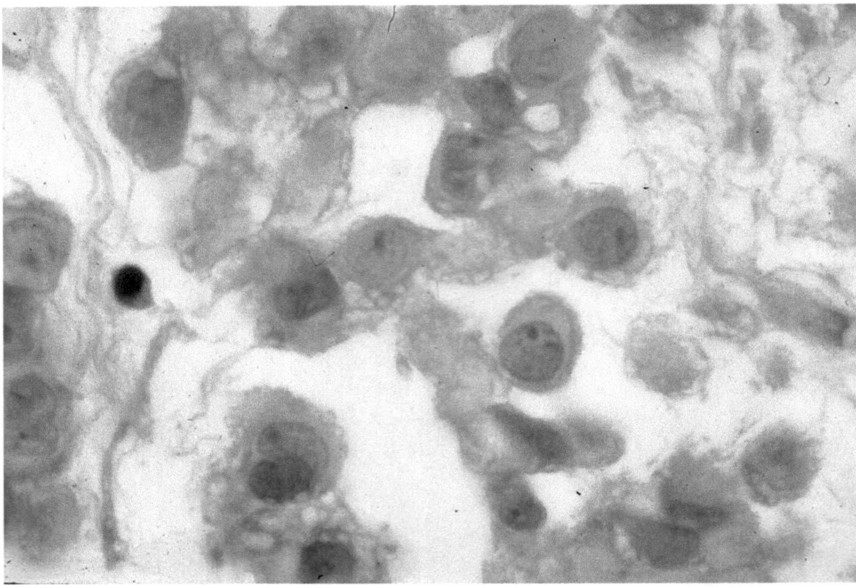

FIGURE 8.49. In this case of mucicarmine positivity, the material present in an extracellular location is eradicated after the tissue has been pretreated with hyaluronidase.

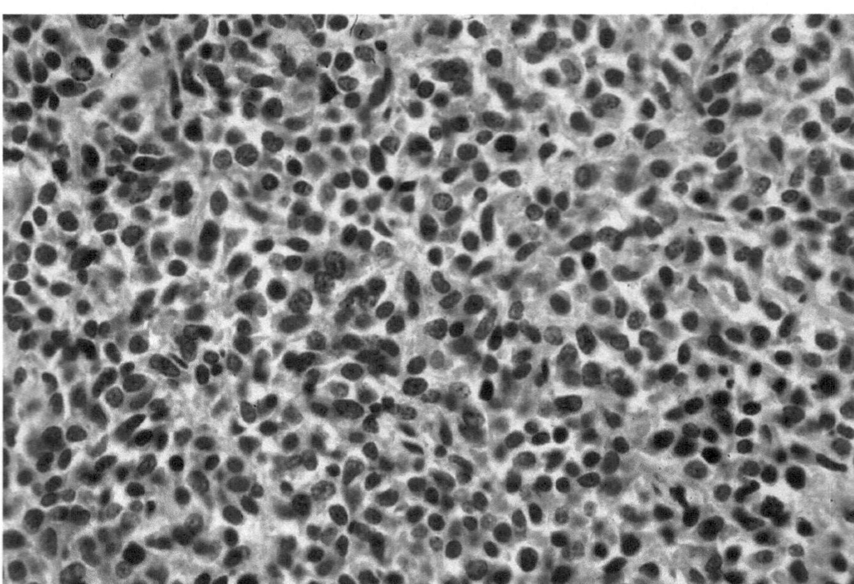

FIGURE 8.50. Mesothelioma composed of small round dark cells.

as the tubulopapillary or glandular variety. The neoplastic small mesothelial cells do not express neuroendocrine markers (CD56, synaptophysin, chromogranin-A) immunohistochemically [35].

Deciduoid mesothelioma was initially reported in the peritoneum of young women and was associated with a poor prognosis, suggesting that it was a specific clinicopathologic entity (Figure 8.51) [36]. The cause of the disease was unknown; and because of the young age of the patients and the failure to demonstrate hormone receptors in the neoplastic cells, it was thought unlikely that asbestos exposure or hormonal imbalance played a role in the development of the disease [36]. Later, and based on the experience of the International Mesothelioma Panel, it was recognized to occur in the pleura of elderly men and women, exhibiting a prognosis similar to that for other types of mesothelioma. The deciduoid appearance is not uncommon as a minor component (Figure 8.52) in more conventional tubulopapillary epithelioid mesotheliomas, but it rarely predominates [37]. In the peritoneum it may be misdiagnosed histologically as a gastrointestinal autonomic nerve tumor (GANT); however, use of immunohistochemical markers such as c-kit (CD117) and cytokeratin should avoid this pitfall [38]. Shia et al. later reported the ultrastructural and clinical findings of five patients with deciduoid mesotheliomas; they demonstrated that the presence of numerous cytoplasmic intermediate filaments, either dispersed or bundled, appeared to be the likely ultrastructural basis for the deciduoid histologic appearance [39].

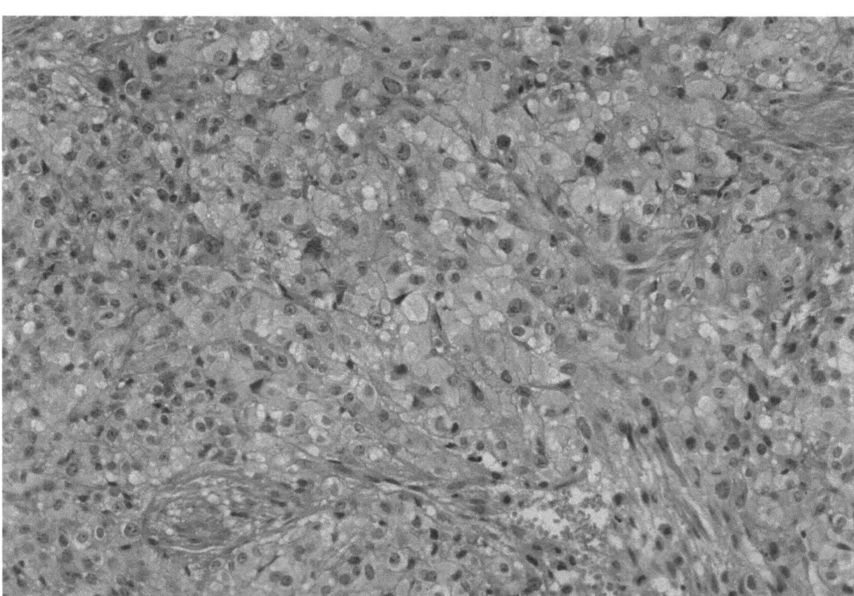

FIGURE 8.51. Epithelioid mesothelioma with diffuse deciduoid appearance.

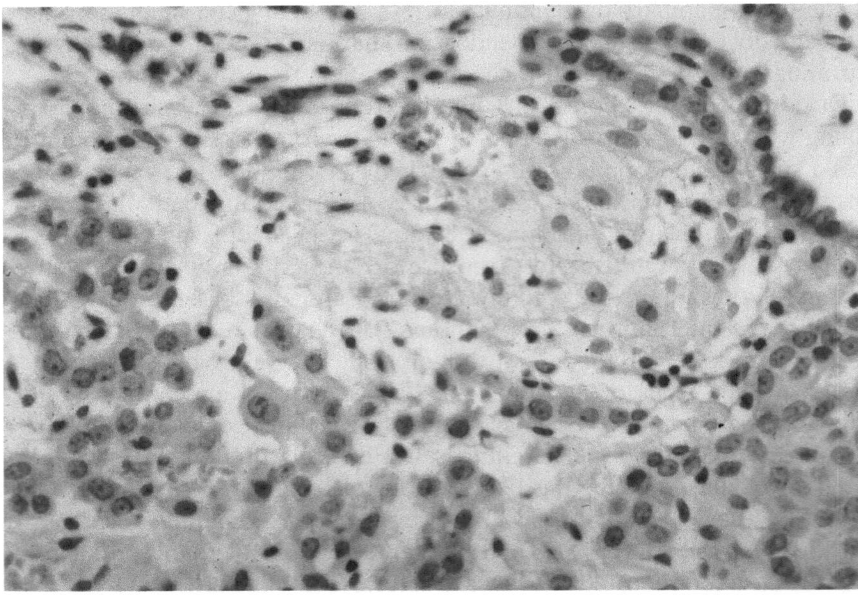

FIGURE 8.52. Deciduoid neoplastic cells mixed with papillary structures seen in a conventional diffuse epithelioid mesothelioma.

The lipid-rich, diffuse malignant mesothelioma is an uncommon epithelioid mesothelioma (Figure 8.53). It is characterized morphologically and ultrastructurally by numerous intracytoplasmic lipid vacuoles and numerous long, branching, and intertwining microvilli characteristic of epithelioid mesothelioma cells [40]. The lesion was first reported by Chang et al. [41]. The lipid vacuoles are useful for separating mesothelial cells from the signet ring cells of adenocarcinoma, which also are PAS-positive and diastase resistant.

Clear cell malignant mesothelioma is an unusual variant that is important to recognize because it may be confused with other metastatic clear cell tumors located to the pleura, especially renal and bronchopulmonary clear cell carcinomas [43, 44] (Figures 8.54–8.56). Immunohistochemistry is extremely useful for reaching the correct diagnosis when the calretinin assay is positive (see below).

The pleomorphic variant of diffuse malignant mesothelioma with spindle and bizarre tumor giant cells shows a histologic resemblance to pleomorphic carcinoma. Calretinin and TTF-1 are useful markers [8] (Figure 8.57).

Differential Diagnosis

The primary differential diagnosis of an epithelioid neoplasm involving the pleura is most commonly between epithelioid mesothelioma and

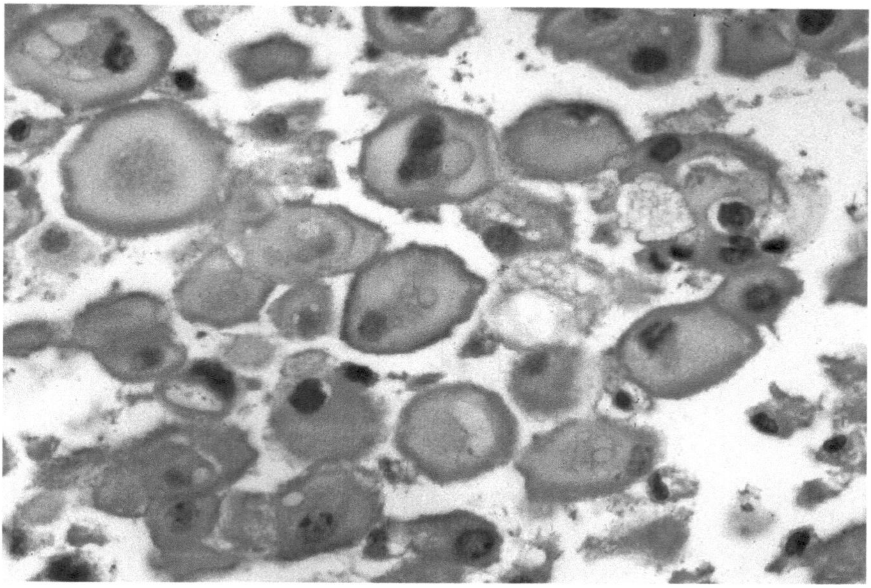

FIGURE 8.53. Lipid-rich diffuse malignant mesothelioma.

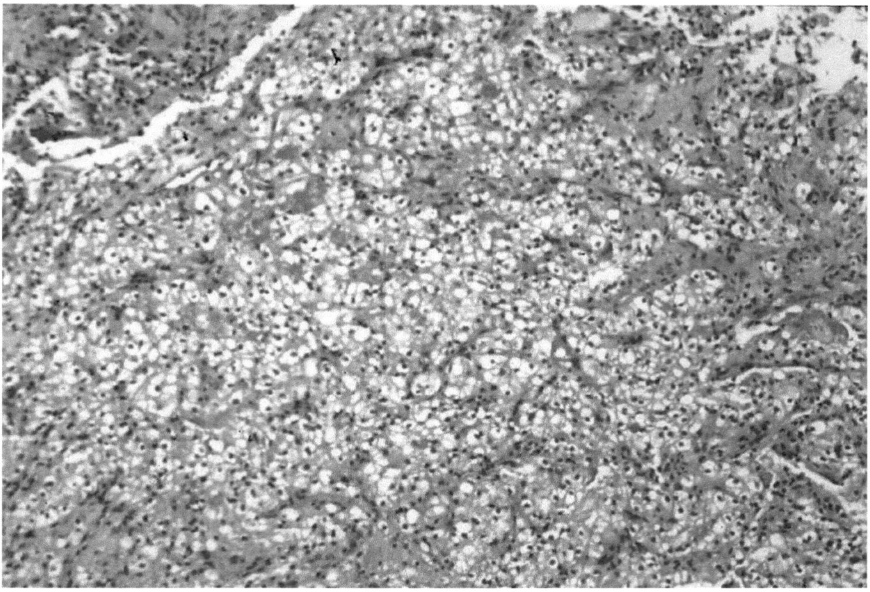

FIGURE 8.54. Low power view of an epithelioid mesothelioma with clear cell features.

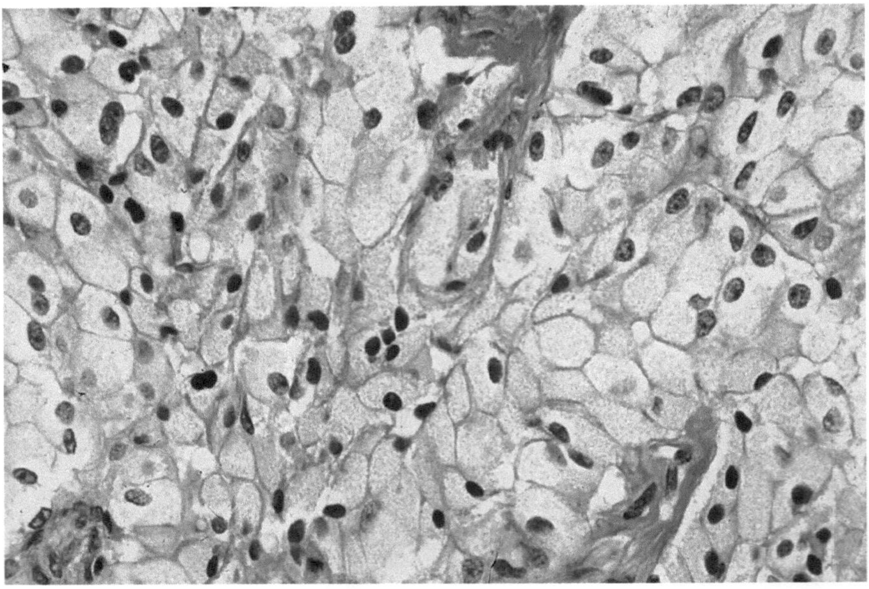

FIGURE 8.55. High power view of clear cell mesothelioma. Note the round, bland central nuclei in contrast with the eccentric nuclei seen in clear cell adenocarcinoma from the kidney.

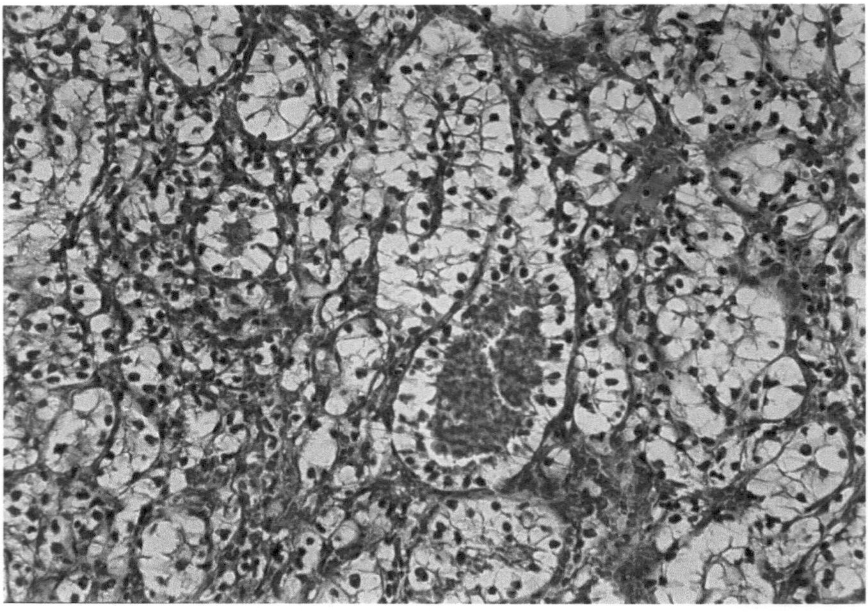

FIGURE 8.56. Renal clear cell carcinoma showing typical glandular structures filled with numerous red blood cells.

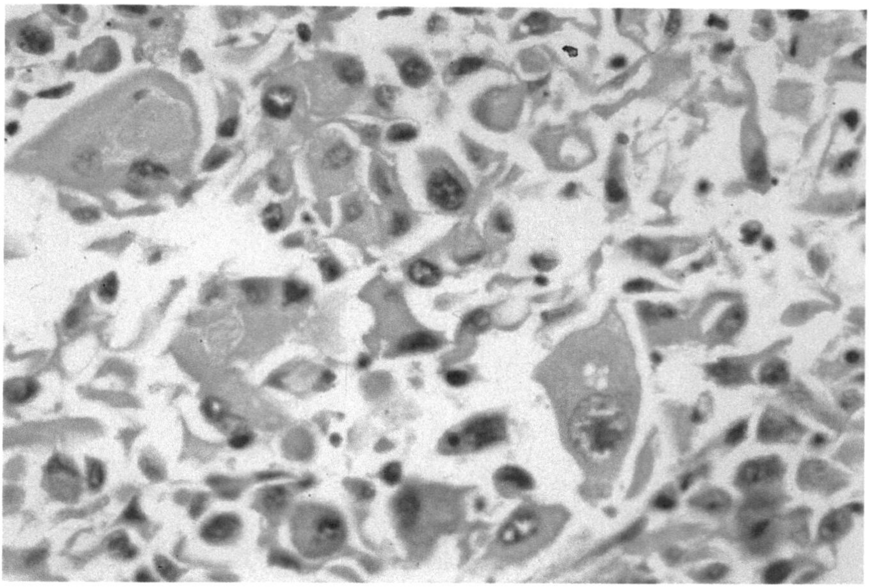

FIGURE 8.57. Pleomorphic mesothelioma with numerous tumor giant cells.

invasive/metastatic pulmonary adenocarcinoma and metastatic adenocarcinoma from an extrathoracic site. It is important to know if there was a history of a prior neoplasm in the patient. These neoplasms can often be differentiated from one another if tissue samples are large enough to perform various immunohistochemical and ultrastructural investigations. If the sample size is small, diagnosis can be difficult and caution is urged.

There is a rare tumor that grows like a mesothelioma and is referred to as a "pseudomesothelioma." Most of these neoplasms are primary pulmonary adenocarcinomas [45, 46], but other histologic types and tumors from other locations may give this appearance. Macroscopically, this tumor may be impossible to differentiate from a primary pleural mesothelioma (Figure 8.58). The most frequent pseudomesotheliomatous adenocarcinoma shows a tubulodesmoplastic pattern in which there are small tubules or glandular structures associated with a large amount of reactive or dense fibrous stromal tissue (Figure 8.59). A significant percentage of these cases are mucin-positive and show immunohistochemical and ultrastructural features of primary pulmonary adenocarcinomas [47–49]. From a practical viewpoint, it usually makes little difference whether a tumor is a mesothelioma or a pseudomesotheliomatous adenocarcinoma. as both have a poor prognosis and in most instances there is no adequate treatment for either neoplasm [45, 47, 49]. They are uncommon, comprising 6% of referrals in the experience of the Environmental Lung Disease Research Group,

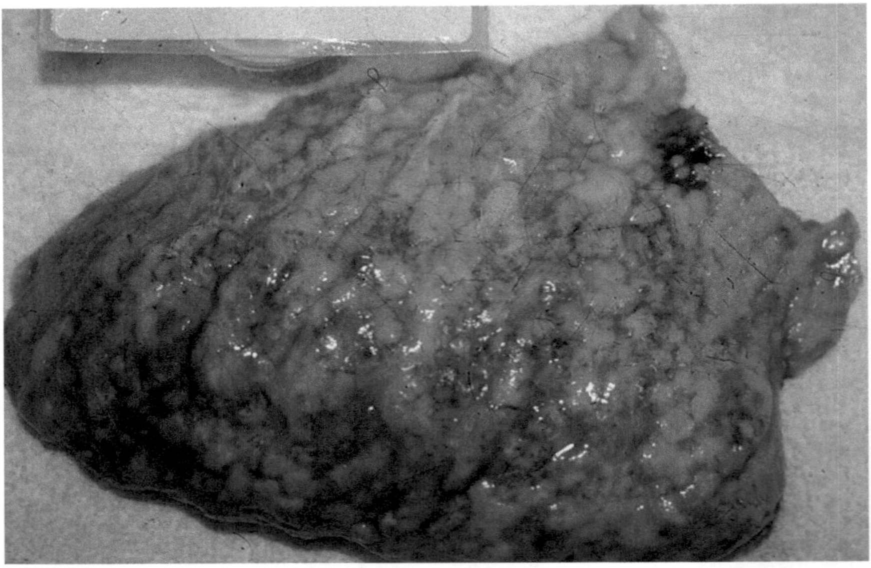

FIGURE 8.58. Diffuse and nodular pleurotropic growth by pseudomesotheliomatous adenocarcinoma.

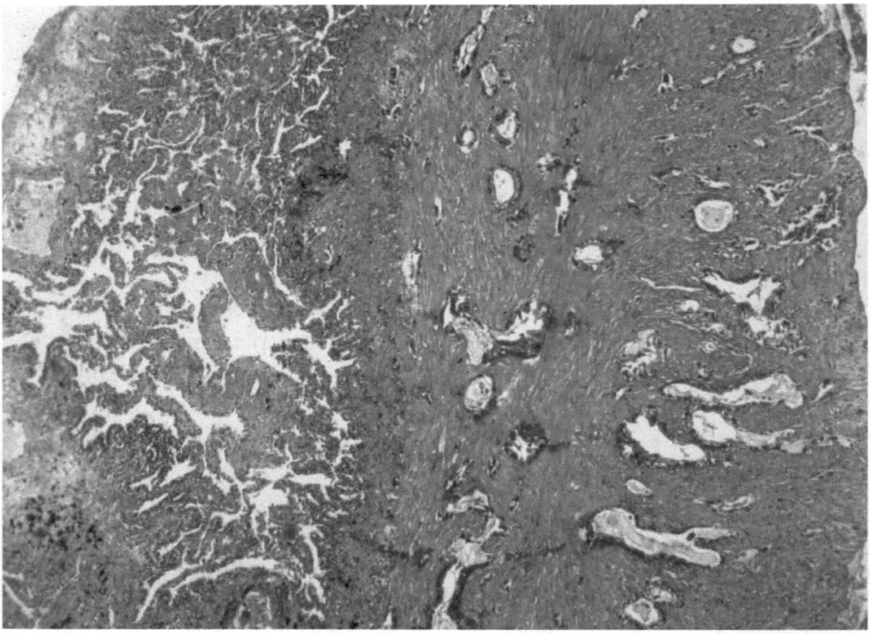

FIGURE 8.59. Pseudomesotheliomatous adenocarcinoma showing prominent fibrous stroma.

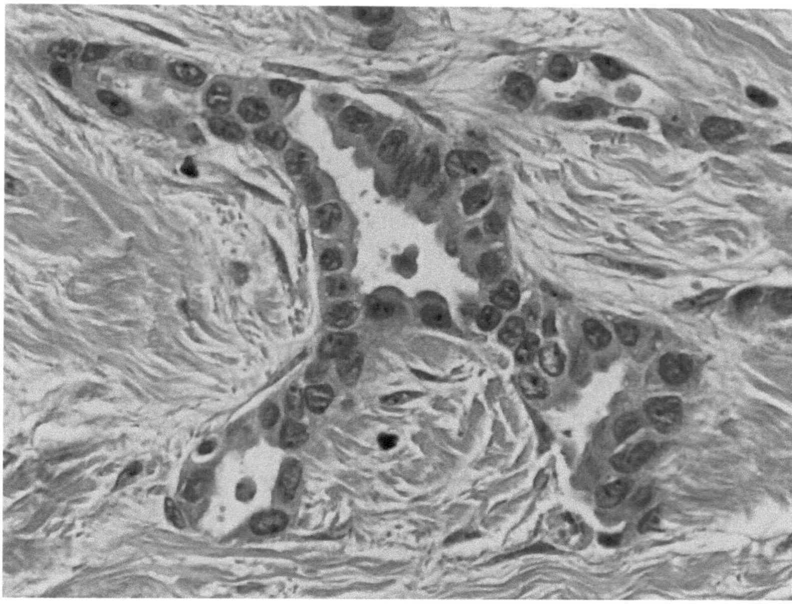

FIGURE 8.60. Pseudomesotheliomatous adenocarcinoma microscopically mimicking epithelioid mesothelioma.

Cardiff [50] and less than 2% in the experience of the French mesothelioma panel (Mesopath Group). Calretinin and TTF-1 are regarded as the most useful markers for the differential diagnosis [51] (Figures 8.60–8.62). Misdiagnosis may have medicolegal implications in asbestos-related compensation claims.

Other neoplasms that may be confused macroscopically and microscopically with pulmonary epithelioid mesothelioma include epithelioid hemangioendothelioma [52, 53] synovial sarcoma [54], intrapleural thymoma [55], melanoma, lymphoma, and a variety of carcinomas [48–50] that are discussed below.

Biphasic Mesothelioma

Biphasic mesothelioma consists of a combined epithelioid and sarcomatoid pattern with the same immunohistochemical pattern seen in the individual components as previously described. The WHO arbitrarily recommended there should be at least 10% of each component present to diagnose biphasic mesothelioma. However, there are no data on the clinical significance of this category and no consensus on these criteria. It is not uncommon for some biphasic mesotheliomas to have a desmoplastic component of less

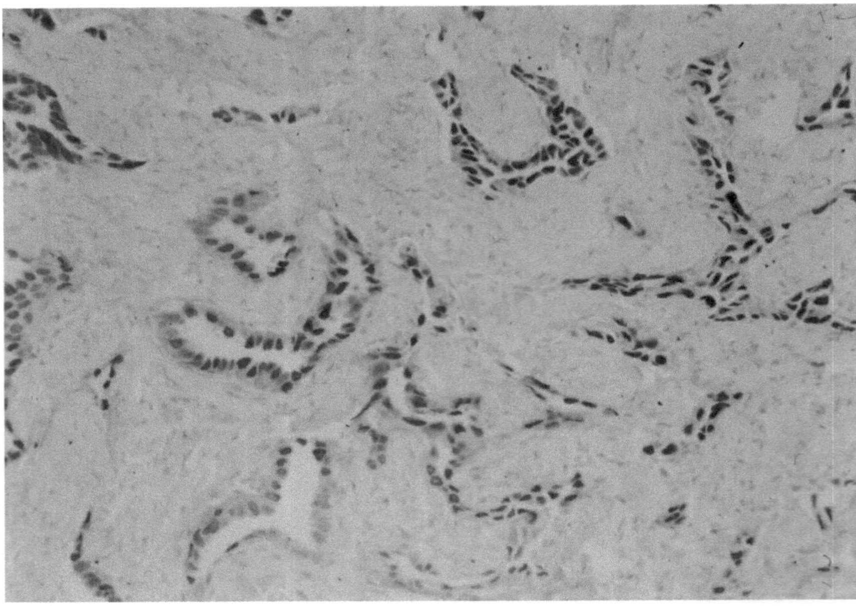

FIGURE 8.61. The same tumor as in Figure 8.60, showing typical intranuclear immunostaining for thyroid transcription factor-1 (TTF-1).

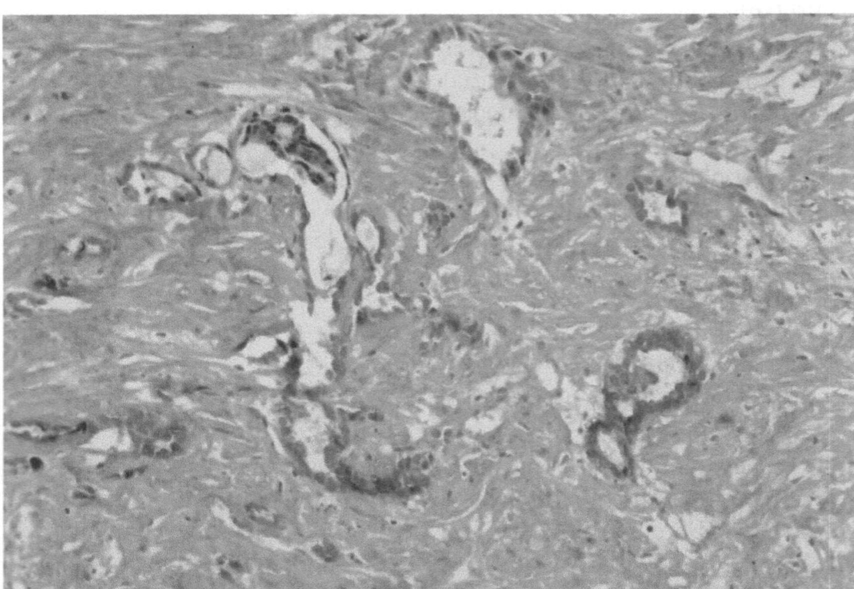

FIGURE 8.62. The same tumor showing cytoplasmic immunostaining for calretinin.

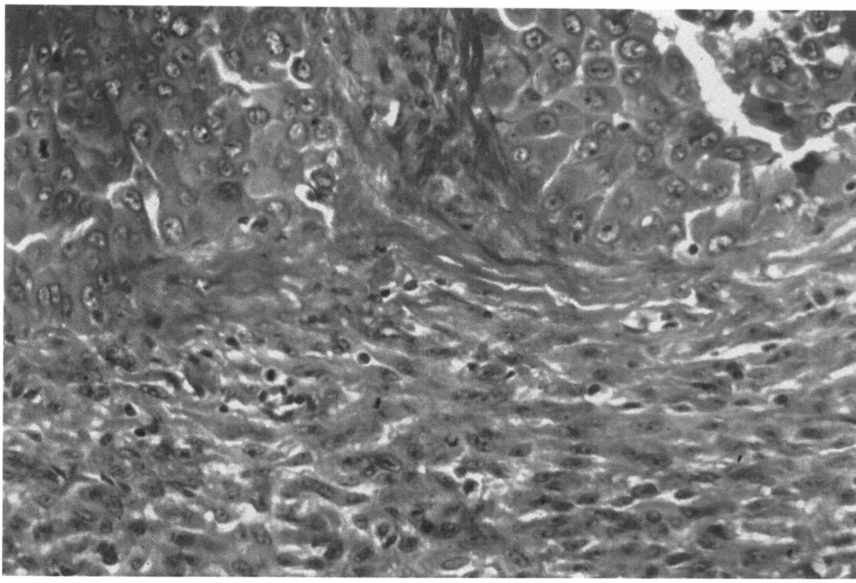

FIGURE 8.63. Biphasic mesothelioma. At the top is a solid sheet of epithelioid cells and at the bottom pleomorphic spindle cells.

than 50%, which can appear extremely benign and can be confused with reactive pleural fibroblastic reactive tissue. From a practical point of view, this is not of any great clinical significance.

It is difficult with some epithelioid mesotheliomas to distinguish reactive stroma from a sarcomatoid component of biphasic mesothelioma. The percentage of mesotheliomas classified as biphasic varies according to location (peritoneum < pleura) [56, 57] and on the extent of sampling. Biphasic mesotheliomas occur in approximatively 30% of patients in various studies and are therefore frequent, especially when a large amount of tissue is available for evaluation such as autopsy tissue or pleuropneumonectomy/radical pleurectomy tissue (Figures 8.63 and 8.64). It is well known that mesotheliomas may show variable degrees of differentiation. We have seen some autopsy mesothelioma specimens in which there were several histologic patterns (Figure 8.65).

Sarcomatoid Mesothelioma

The sarcomatoid variant of mesothelioma accounts for about 10% to 20% of pleural cases but less than 4% of peritoneal cases. These tumors may present as nodules or confluent lesions without pleural effusion. Rarely,

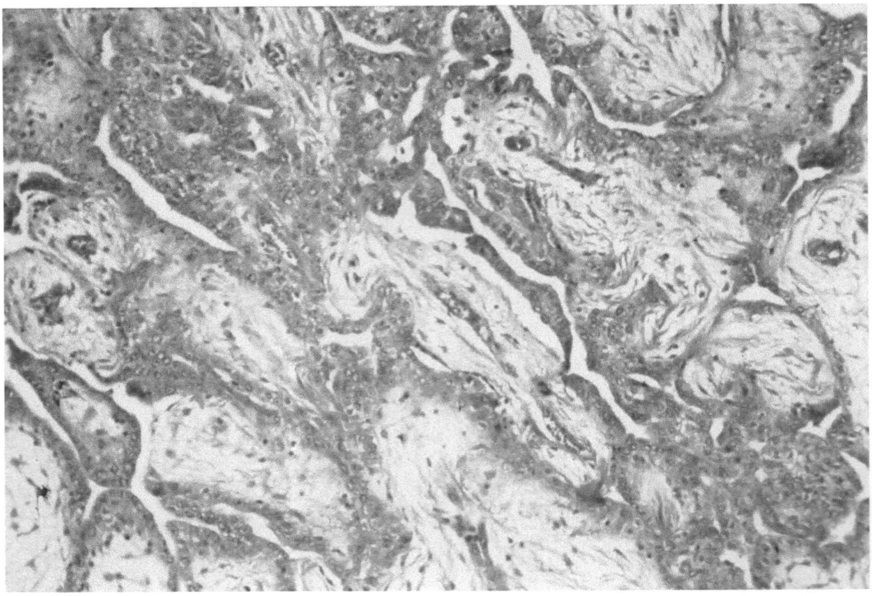

FIGURE 8.64. Epithelioid mesothelioma composed of tubules and papillae with prominent hypercellular reactive stroma mimicking a biphasic tumor.

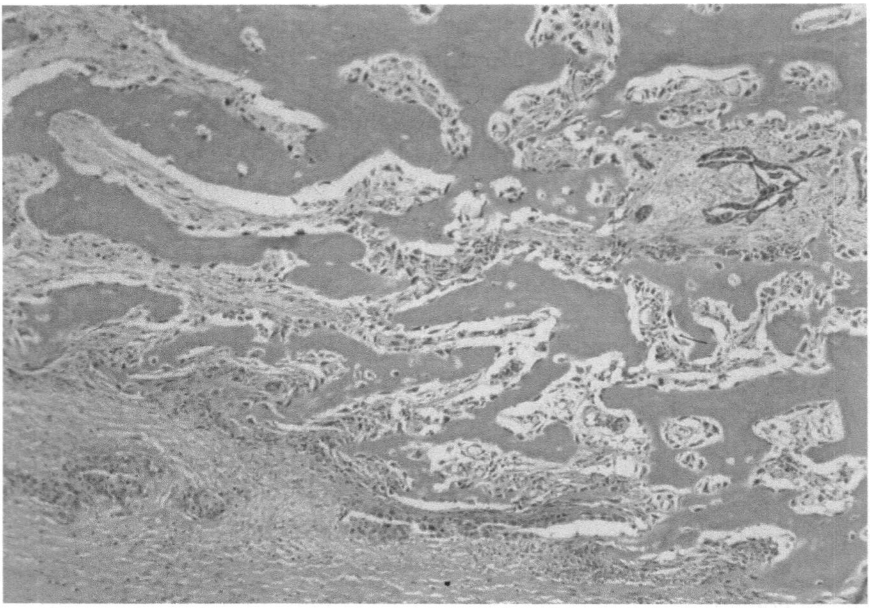

FIGURE 8.65. Biphasic mesothelioma showing tubular and osteocartilaginous differentiation.

they present as a localized pleural mass [58–61]. Surgical dissection Dissection of such cases is extremely difficult because of chest wall invasion and the rigid nature of the tumor. In the peritoneum the tumor frequently encases abdominal viscera, making identification of a gastrointestinal or genitourinary primary tumor difficult if not impossible.

Histologic Examination

Sarcomatoid mesotheliomas consist of a pure spindled pattern resembling that of a fibrosarcoma or a malignant fibrous histiocytoma [1, 61, 62]. These tumors have also been called sarcomatous, spindled, and diffuse malignant fibrous mesothelioma. They typically consist of spindle cells arranged haphazardly or in fascicles. At low magnification, nodules of tumor infiltrate surrounding tissues, including parietal pleural fat. The nuclei are elongated to plump, and nucleoli may be prominent (Figure 8.66). Necrosis and mitotic activity are variable. The tumor cells may be surrounded by collagen or myxoid stroma. Chronic inflammation is usually minimal. These tumors most often resemble fibrosarcoma (Figure 8.66), but marked anaplasia and bizarre multinucleate tumor cells may result in a pattern closely mimicking malignant fibrous histiocytoma (Figure 8.67). In a small per-

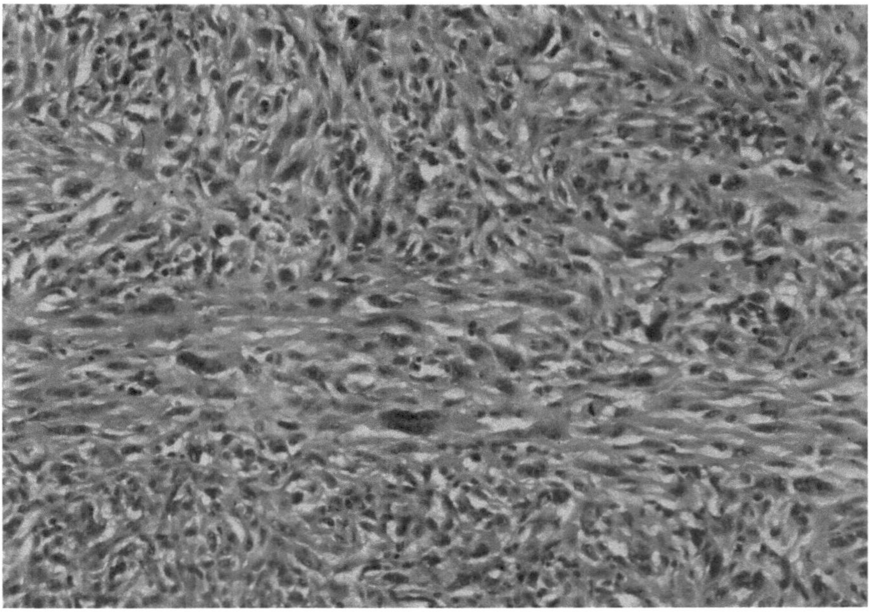

FIGURE 8.66. Sarcomatoid pleural mesothelioma showing fascicles of atypical spindle cells with hyperchromatic nuclei.

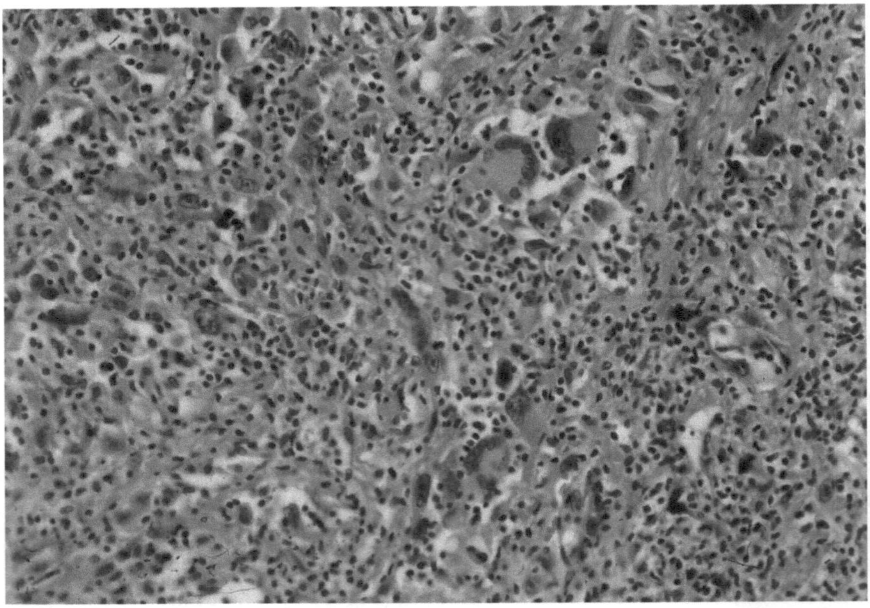

FIGURE 8.67. Sarcomatoid pleural mesothelioma showing bizarre anaplastic tumor giant cells. Such an appearance closely mimics that of malignant fibrous histiocytoma.

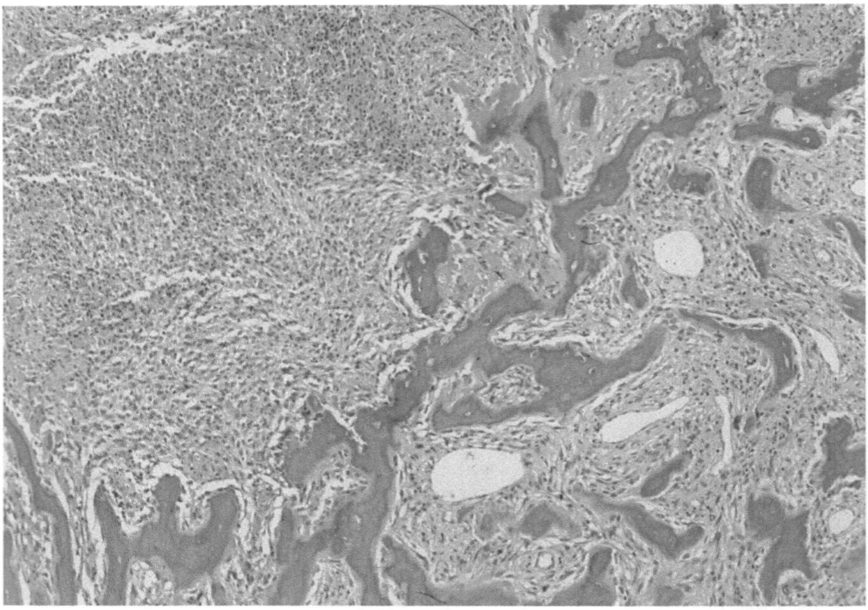

FIGURE 8.68. Sarcomatoid mesothelioma with osteosarcomatous differentiation showing spicules of bone or osteoid produced by the tumor.

centage of cases, areas resembling osteosarcoma or chondrosarcoma, leiomyosarcoma, and rhabdomyosarcoma may be present (Figure 8.68) [63, 64]. In some cases, these areas are so prominent that calcified densities can be seen within the tumor radiographically (Figure 8.69). Other forms of sarcomatous differentiation potentially can occur in mesotheliomas, but they are not well documented.

Sarcomatoid mesotheliomas must be distinguished from organizing fibrous pleuritis, localized fibrous tumors of the serous membranes (LFTs), sarcomatoid carcinomas, primary and metastatic sarcomas involving the pleura, and desmoid tumors. Histologic features and cytokeratin staining can help exlude LFTs, desmoid tumors, and metastatic sarcomas.

Gross features are also useful, as LFTs and desmoid tumors present as a localized pleura-based mass, and metastatic sarcomas tend to present as multiple pleural based nodules. However, the differentiation from sarcomatoid (pleomorphic) carcinoma of the lung secondarily invading the pleura or metastatic sarcomatoid mammary or renal cell carcinoma can be exceedingly difficult. Immunostains do not reliably differentiate between these diagnostic possibilities, as all of these tumors are typically keratin-positive and negative for glycoprotein markers [65]. In such cases, the gross features can be helpful. A diagnosis of sarcomatoid mesothelioma should

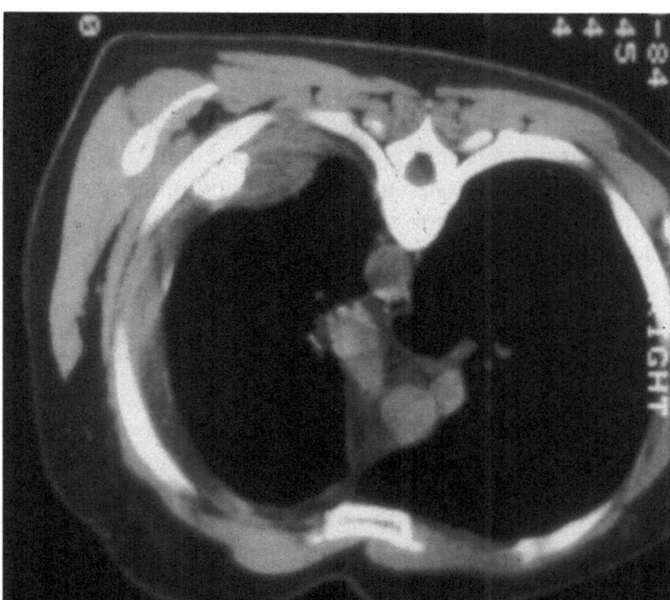

FIGURE 8.69. Computed tomographic scan of the thorax in a patient with osteosarcomatous variant of pleural mesothelioma. Note the calcific density within the tumor mass.

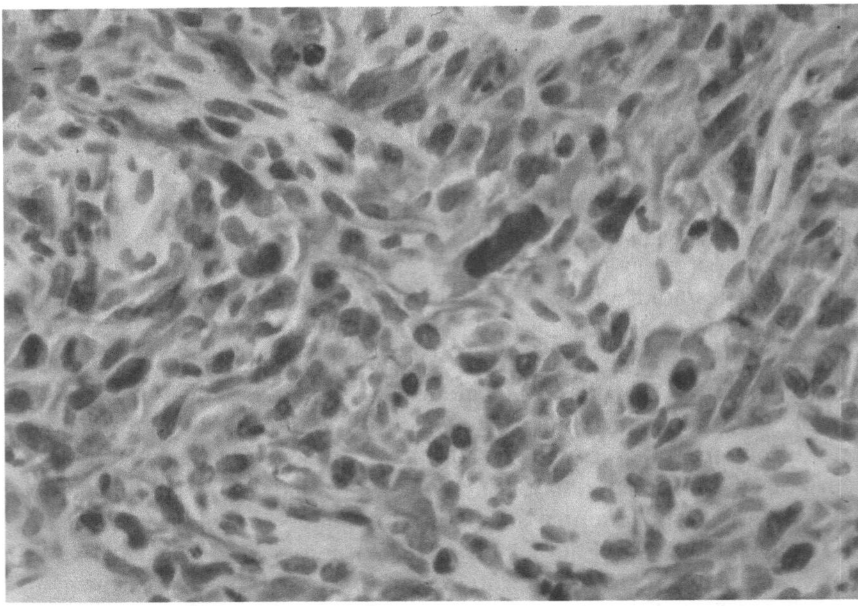

FIGURE 8.70. Immunohistochemical staining of a sarcomatoid mesothelioma for cytokeratins, showing diffuse cytoplasmic positivity in virtually all tumor cells.

be made with great caution in a patient with a radiologic lung mass, as it often represents a sarcomatoid or pleomorphic carcinoma of the lung. Similarly, caution should be used when diagnosing a pleural mesothelioma in a patient with a known renal mass, as renal cell carcinomas (including sarcomatoid variants) can metastasize to the pleura and mimic a mesothelioma. In such instances, mesothelioma should only be diagnosed when both the renal and pleural tumor have been sampled and shown to be histologically dissimilar.

Immunohistochemical Features

Histochemical stains are not helpful in the differential diagnosis of sarcomatoid mesotheliomas because acid mucopolysaccharides are present in the stroma of any soft tissue sarcoma. However, immunohistochemical stains for cytokeratins are useful in the diagnosis of these neoplasms. In the typical case, the tumor cells stain strongly and are diffusely positive with a cocktail containing antibodies to both high- and low-molecular-weight cytokeratins (e.g., AE_1/AE_3 and Cam 5.2) (Figure 8.70). Variable staining for cytokeratins may be seen, with strong staining in some areas of the tumor and absence of staining in other areas. In perhaps 10% or fewer sar-

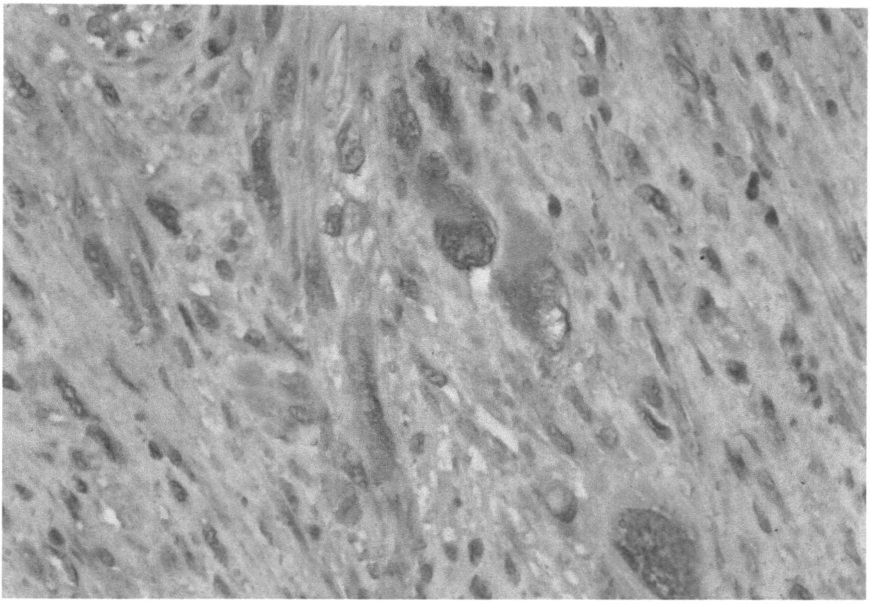

FIGURE 8.71. Immunohistochemical staining of a sarcomatoid mesothelioma for calretinin showing nuclear positivity in many tumor cells.

comatoid mesotheliomas, there is an absence of staining for cytokeratins. For this reason, a cocktail should be used. In such exceptional cases, the diagnosis rests on typical gross distribution and histologic findings and exclusion of a primary sarcoma elsewhere. Interestingly, areas with chondrosarcomatous or osteosarcomatous differentiation often stain negatively for cytokeratins [63, 64]. Sarcomatoid mesotheliomas are usually positive for vimentin, which is a useful marker for the adequacy of the fixation. They may also stain positively for actin and desmin or S-100. Some 20% of cases also show focal nuclear staining for calretinin (Figure 8.71) or CK5/6 [65].

Electron Microscopic Features

Ultrastructurally, sarcomatoid mesotheliomas have features similar to those of fibroblasts or myofibroblasts. The stroma consists primarily of collagen fibers (Figure 8.72). Adjacent tumor cells may be connected by intermediate-type junctions. In some cases, the spindle-shaped tumor cells contain tonofilaments and exhibit a few surface microvilli. True desmosomes may also be noted in such instances. In the absence of the latter findings, the ultrastructural features of sarcomatoid mesotheliomas are nonspecific [66].

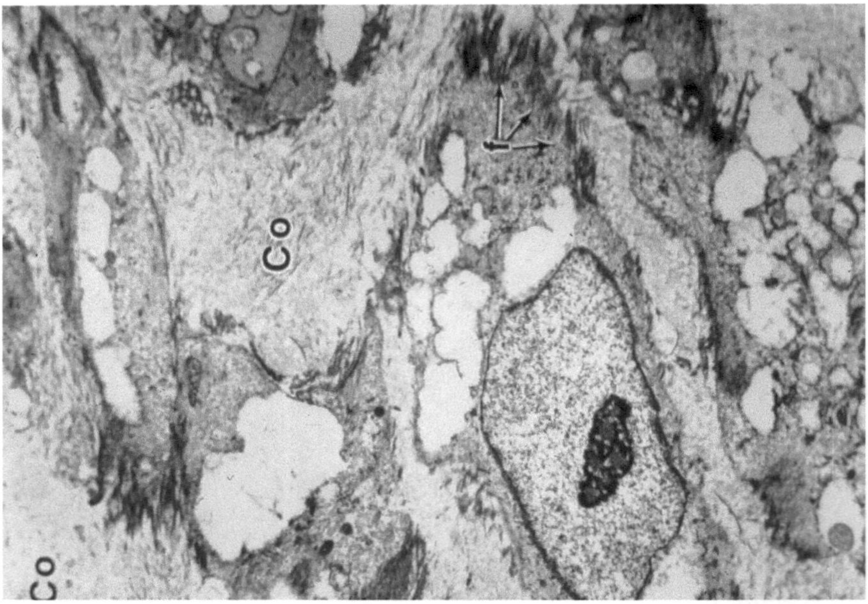

FIGURE 8.72. Transmission electron micrograph of sarcomatoid mesothelioma, showing spindle cells with features of fibroblasts or myofibroblasts. There is abundant extracellular collagen.

Desmoplastic Malignant Mesothelioma

According to the 2004 WHO classification [67], desmoplastic mesothelioma is a sarcomatoid mesothelioma with a predominance (>50%) of dense collagenous stroma and haphazardly arranged slit-like spaces made up of cells with slightly atypical nuclei (Figures 8.73–8.75). Most of these tumors originate in the pleura, but such tumors arising in the peritoneum have been described (Figure 8.76) [68, 69]. Most tumors are sarcomatoid, but some desmoplastic mesotheliomas with a biphasic or even an epithelioid component have been reported. In the French series (1998–2002) of 709 consecutive mesotheliomas published in the annual report of activities of the Programme National de Surveillance des Mésothéliomes (PNSM) to the Institut de Veille Sanitaire (INVS), desmoplastic variants accounted for about 2% of cases [70].

Because of the abundant fibrous tissue separating scattered neoplastic cells, these tumors can readily be confused with fibrous pleurisy. Invasion of lung parenchyma may also resemble organizing pneumonia. Large biopsies are preferable. The reader should be aware that a surface empyema possibly due to needling can occur in combination with a malignant mesothelioma underneath. In desmoplastic malignant mesotheliomas (DMMs), all biopsy tissue must be processed and levels cut if necessary. The

FIGURE 8.73. Low power view of desmoplastic malignant mesothelioma. There is a subtle change in color in the transition from largely collagenized areas of tumor (pink) to the more cellular areas (blue).

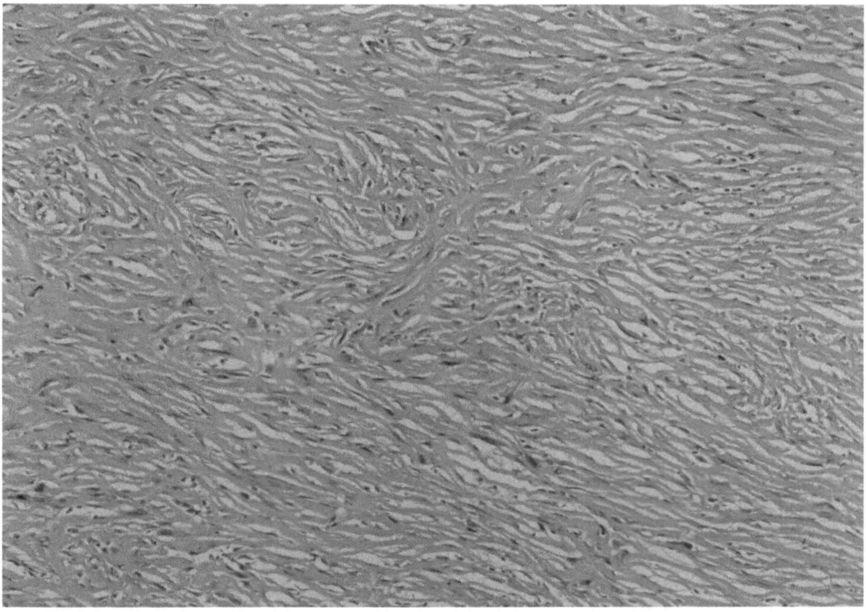

FIGURE 8.74. Less cellular areas of the tumor in Figure 8/73, showing band of collagen arranged in the "patternless pattern" of Stout, separated by hyperchromatic tumor nuclei.

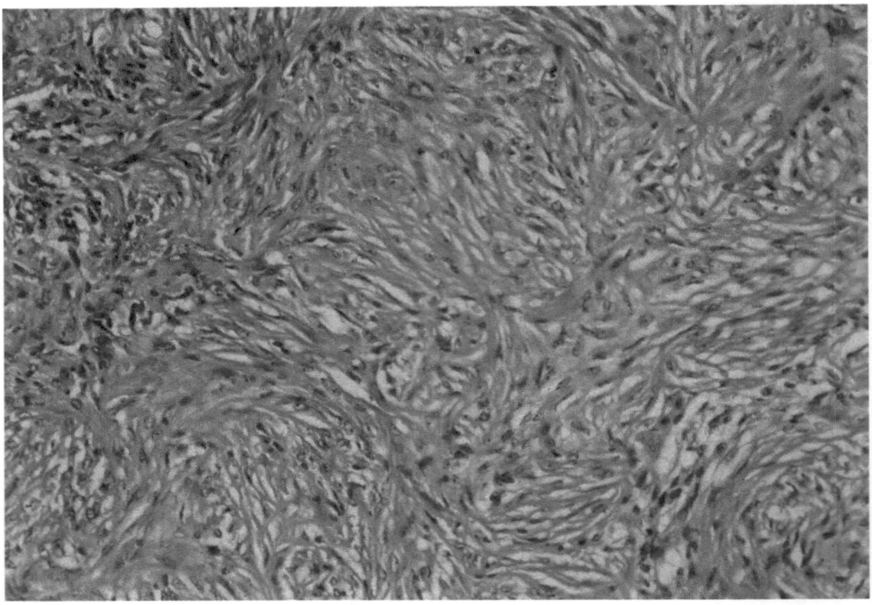

FIGURE 8.75. More cellular area of the tumor in Figure 8.73 shows atypical spindle cells arranged in a storiform pattern.

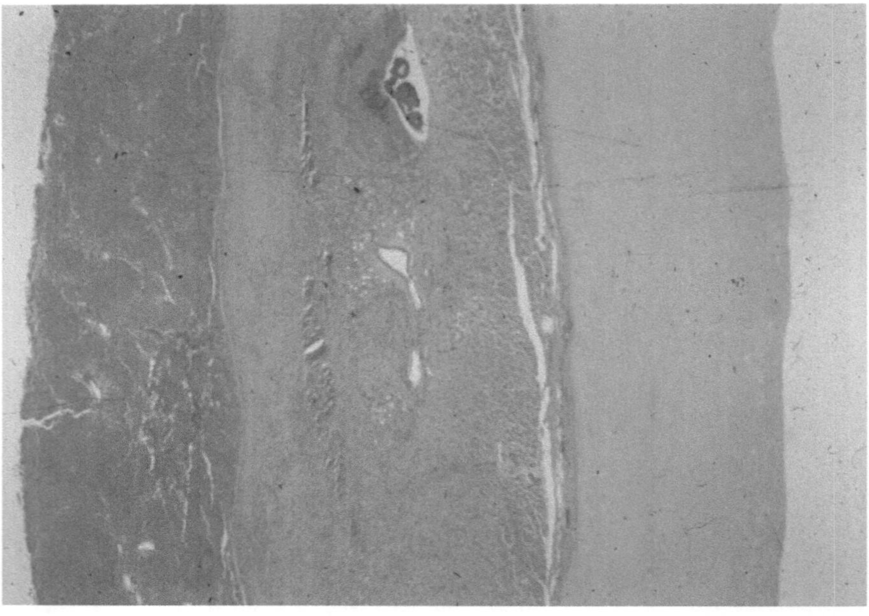

FIGURE 8.76. Low power view of a desmoplastic malignant mesothelioma localized to the lower pleural cavity. Distinct layers are seen from the right to the left consisting of parietal pleural plaque and mesothelioma.

diagnosis is especially difficult and should be made circumspectly from a closed needle biopsy specimen. However, there are certain diagnostic criteria that strongly suggest a diagnosis of malignancy. These findings include frankly sarcomatoid areas; foci of bland necrosis; invasion of adipose tissue, skeletal muscle, or lung; and distant metastases [71]. The tumor may grow as nodular expansile masses on a background of reactive pleuritis. Frankly sarcomatoid areas are recognized as regions of more intense cellularity, with a patternless pattern or focal storifom foci. The atypical spindle cells have atypical, often hyperchromatic nuclei (Figure 8.77). Mitotic figures are variable. There is often an abrupt transition from relatively acellular to more hypercellular regions. Areas of bland necrosis appear as subtle areas of altered staining that on higher magnification are seen to contain nuclear debris but no or little inflammation. These foci of necrosis may be associated with vascular invasion and thrombus in a central vessel (Figure 8.78).

Invasion of adipose tissue, skeletal muscle, or lung as well as metastasis are important criteria of malignancy (Figures 8.79–8.82). Ancillary studies are of limited utililty in the differential diagnosis of DMM. Cytokeratin staining may be of greatest utility by highlighting invasion of keratin-positive spindle cells in adipose tissue and skeletal muscle [Figures 8.83, 8.84). The mere presence of keratin-positive staining is of no particular benefit because reactive processes often have keratin-positive spindle cells. Immunostaining of more than 10% of spindle cell nuclei for p53 is

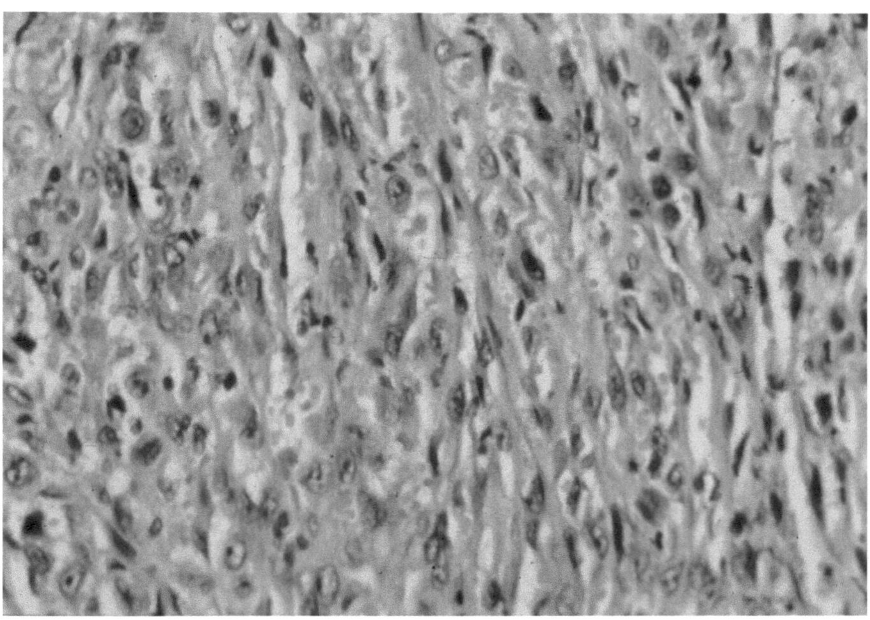

FIGURE 8.77. Frankly sarcomatoid focus in a desmoplastic malignant mesothelioma, showing prominent cellularity and nuclear anaplasia.

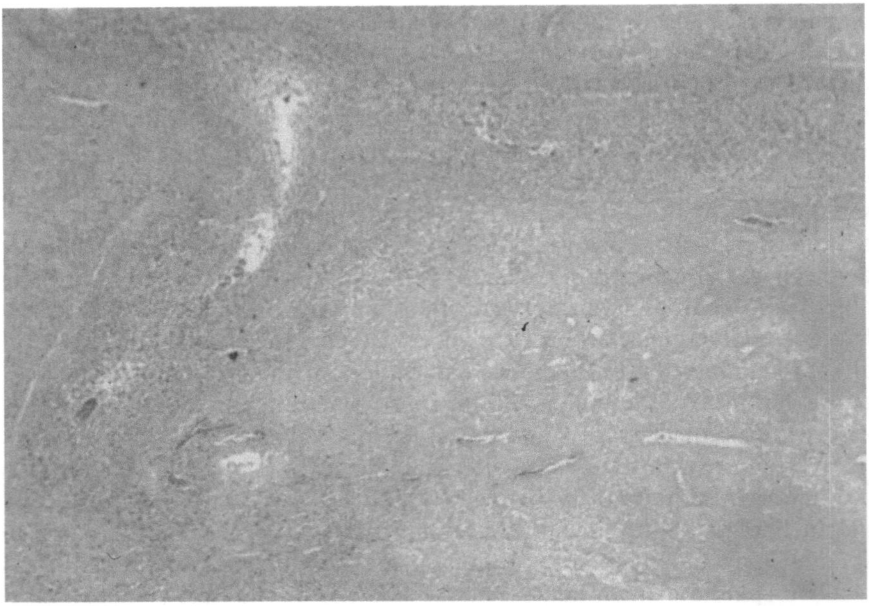

FIGURE 8.78. Focus of bland necrosis in a desmoplastic mesothelioma, showing subtle changes in staining characteristics in the necrotic area. Note invasion of the blood vessel by tumor in the upper part.

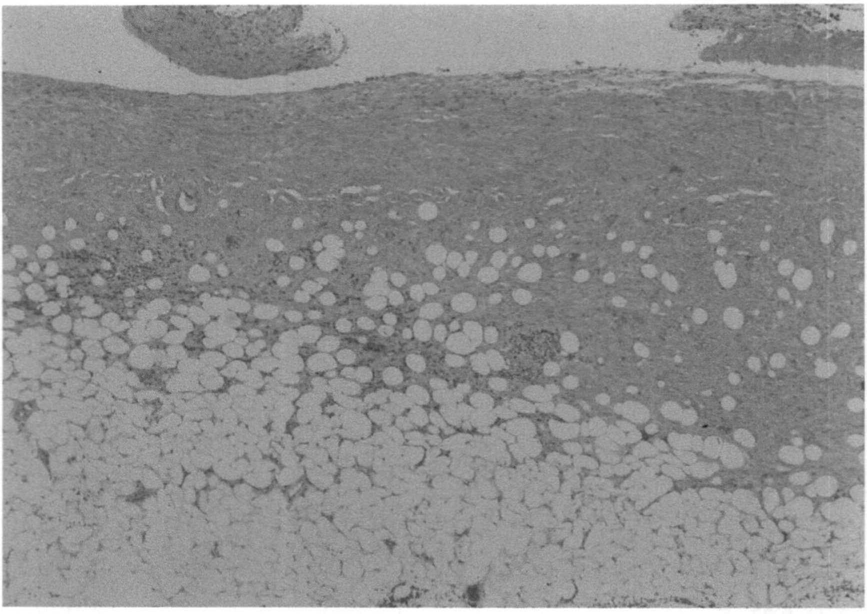

FIGURE 8.79. Invasion of adipose tissue of the chest wall by desmoplastic mesothelioma.

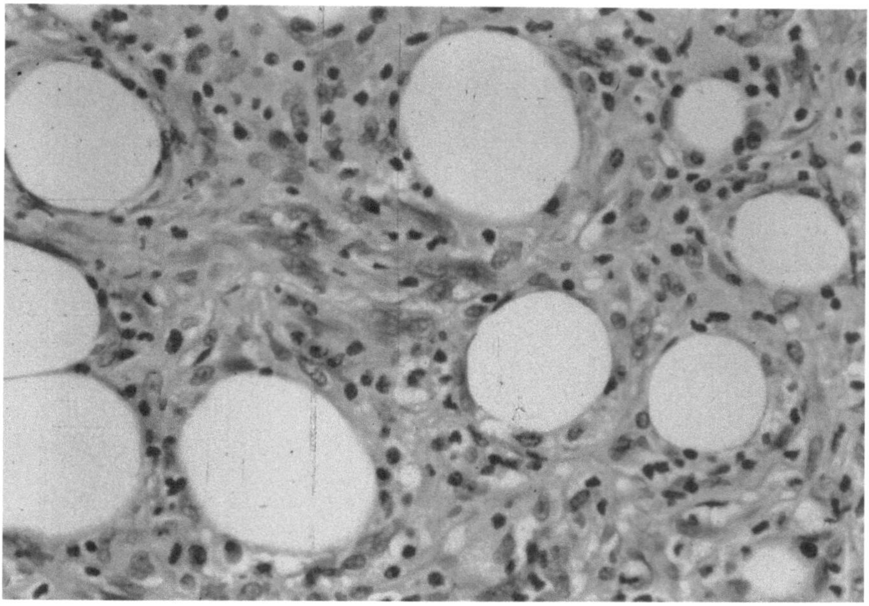

FIGURE 8.80. Higher magnification of a different case from that in Figure 8.79, showing invasion of adipose tissue. Note the insinuation of neoplastic spindle cells between individual fat cells.

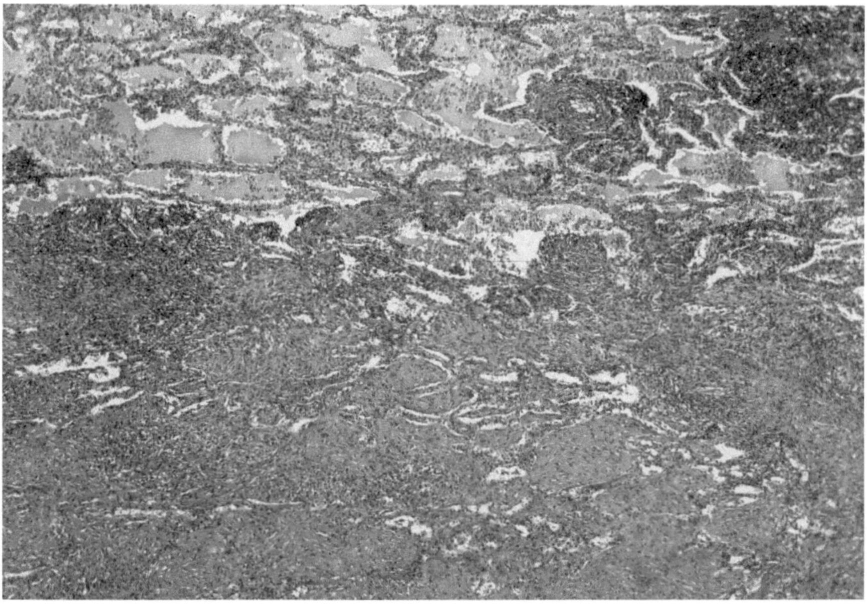

A

FIGURE 8.81. A. Low power view showing invasion of lung tissue by desmoplastic mesothelioma, with a superficial resemblance to organizing pneumonia. B. High power view showing invasion of lung tissue by the desmoplastic mesothelioma.

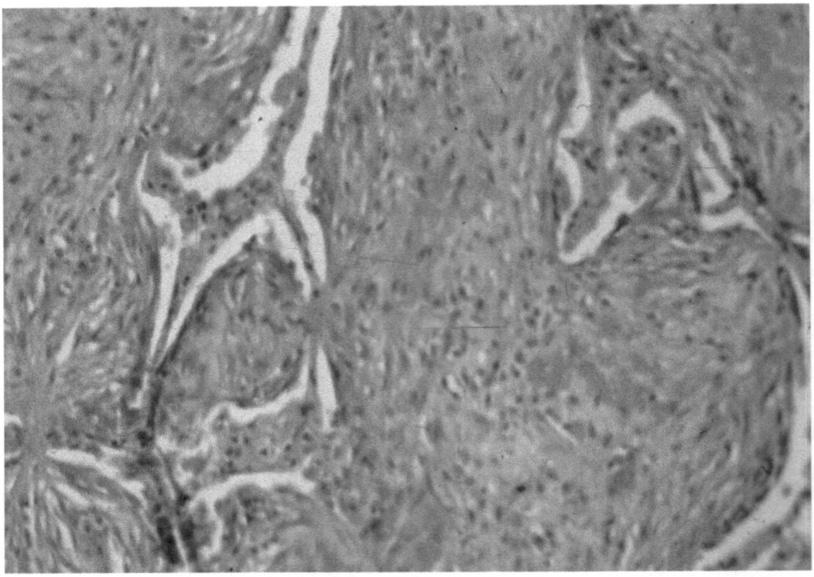

B

FIGURE 8.81. *Continued*

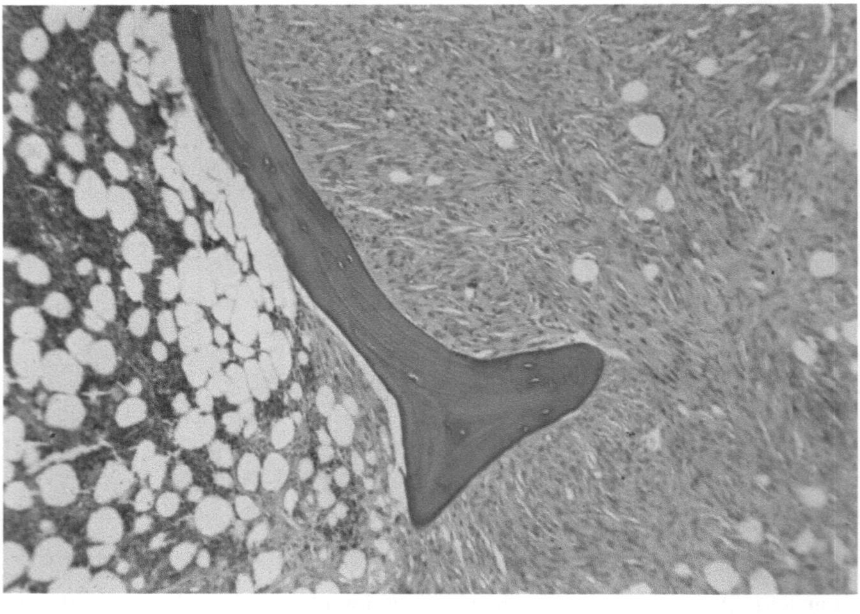

FIGURE 8.82. Metastatic deposit of desmoplastic malignant mesothelioma in bone.

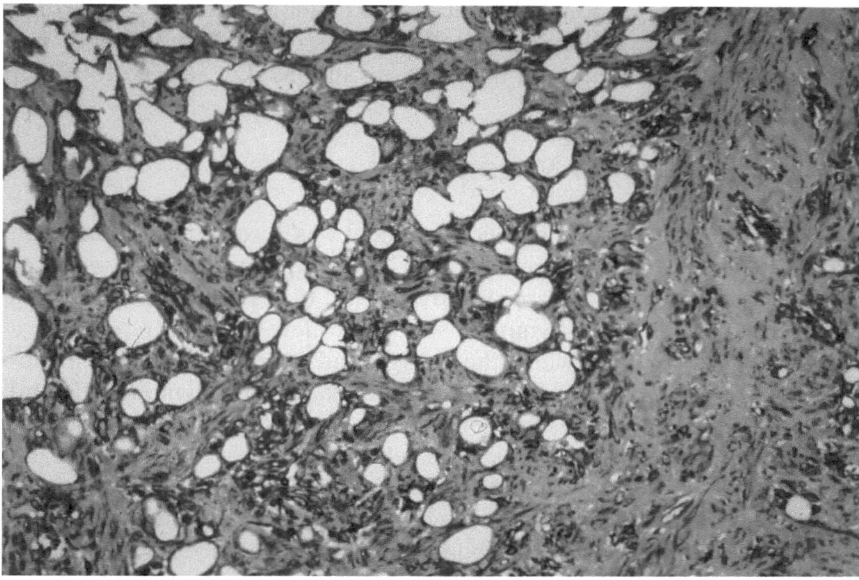

FIGURE 8.83. Cytokeratin immunostaining highlights the invasion of neoplastic spindle cells in adipose tissue.

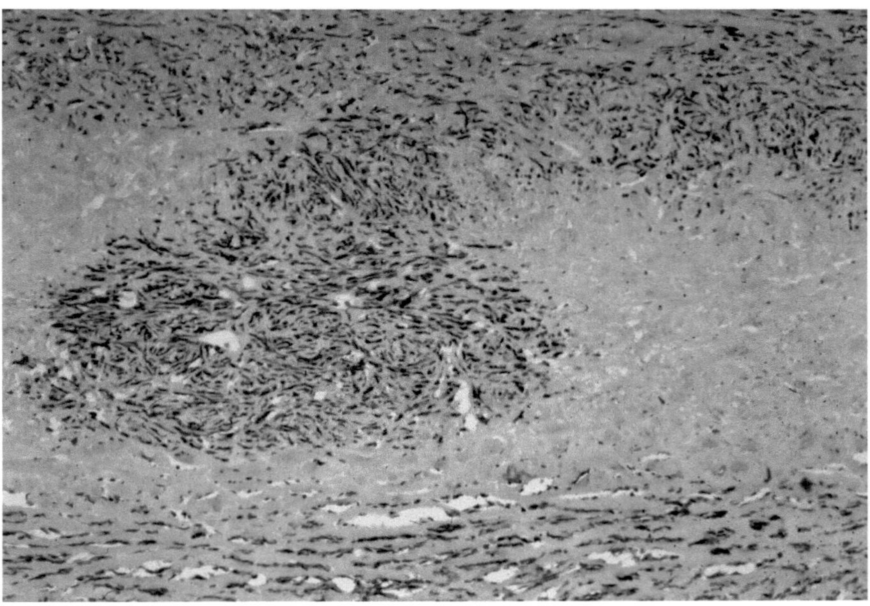

FIGURE 8.84. Cytokeratin positivity highlighting a nest of proliferation in a desmoplastic mesothelioma.

suggestive of DMM, although this finding has no more predictive value than the histologic findings alone [69, 71, 72]. Ultrastructural studies have not been shown to be of benefit in the diagnosis of DMM.

Lymphohistiocytoid Mesothelioma

The lymphohistiocytoid mesothelioma variant was described by Henderson et al. in 1988 [73] and by Khalidi et al. in 2000 [74]. A series of 21 cases was reported in 2003 by the Mesopath Group [75]. It is a rare entity occuring in less than 2% of cases. Lymphohistiocytoid mesothelioma represents a form of mesothelioma in which the background neoplastic cells are histiocytoid in appearance, arranged in nests admixed with a lymphocytic and plasma cell infiltrate. The histiocytoid cells co-express cytokeratin, vimentin, calretinin, and CK5/6. The histiocytoid cells are negative for lymphoid and macrophages markers. By analogy with the criteria for the diagnosis of desmoplastic mesothelioma, it is suggested that 50% of the tumor or more in a biopsy sample should be lymphoma-like in appearance for a diagnosis of lymphohistiocytoid mesothelioma to be made.

The original criterion for recognizing this form of mesothelioma was that each case was misdiagnosed at some time as serous-based lymphoma (Figure 8.85). Epithelioid mesotheliomas with a prominent stromal lym-

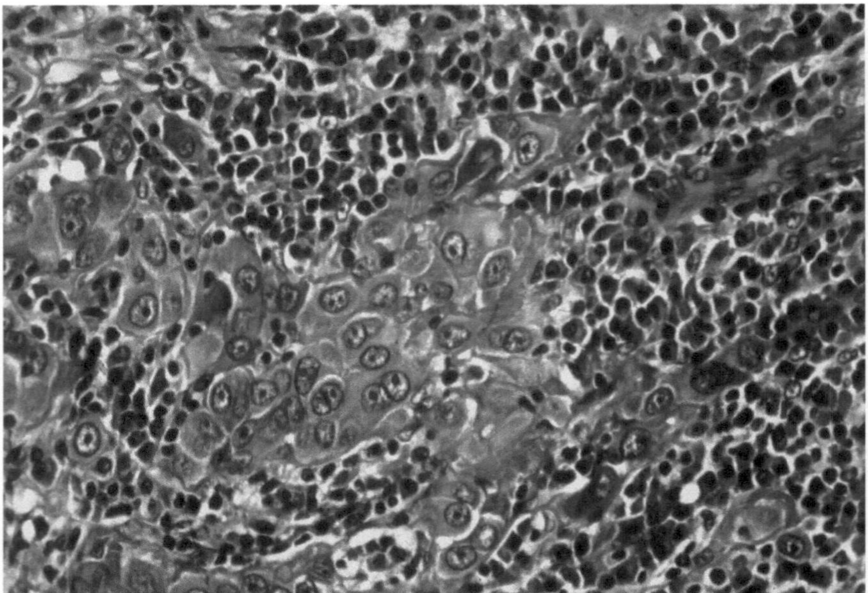

FIGURE 8.85. Lymphohistiocytoid mesothelioma showing numerous lymphoid cells in association with large epithelioid mesothelial cells mimicking lymphoma.

phoid infiltrate do not represent lymphohistiocytoid mesotheliomas. They also are misdiagnosed as lymphoepithelial–like carcinoma reaching the pleura or as pleura-based thymic epithelial tumors [76]. AE1/AE3 and calretinin, are important discriminatory assays. The tumor is not related to Epstein-Barr virus infection, as it stains negatively for for LMP1 and EBER-1 by, respectively, immunohistochemical and in situ hybridization analysis.

References

1. Travis WD, Colby TV, Corrin B, et al. Histological typing of lung and pleural tumors, 3rd edition. Geneva: WHO; 1999.
2. Churg A. Neoplastic asbestos induced disease. In: Churg A, Green FHY (eds). Pathology of occupational lung disease, 2nd edition. Baltimore: Williams & Wilkins; 1998:356.
3. Hammar SP. Pleural diseases. In: Dail DH, Hammar SP (eds) Pulmonary pathology. New York: Springer-Verlag; 1993:1463.
4. Attanoos RL, Gibbs AR. Pathology of malignant mesothelioma. Histopathology 1997;30:413–8.
5. Hasleton PS. Pleural disease. In: Haslton PS (ed) Spencer's pathology of the lung, 5th edition. New York: McGraw-Hill: 1996:1131.
6. Nascimento GA, Keeney GL, Fletcher CD. Deciduoid peritoneal mesothelioma: an unusual phenotype affecting young females. Am J Surg Pathol 1994;18:439–45.
7. Shanks JH, Harris M, Banerjee SS, et al. Mesotheliomas with deciduoid morphology: a morphologic spectrum and a variant not confined to young females. Am J Surg Pathol 2000;24:285–94.
8. Riera JR, Astengo-Osuana C, Longmate JA, et al. The immunohistochemical diagnostic panel for epithelial mesothelioma: a reevaluation after heat-induced epitope retrieval. Am J Surg Pathol 1997;21:1409–19.
9. Carella R, Deleonardi G, D'Errico A. et al. Immunohistochemical panels for differentiating epithelial malignant mesothelioma from lung adenocarcinoma: a study with logistic regression analysis. Am J Surg Pathol 2001;25:43–50.
10. Ordonnez N. The immunohistochemical diagnosis of mesothelioma: a comparative study of epithelioid mesothelioma and lung adenocarcinoma. Am J Surg Pathol 2003;27:1031–51.
11. Miettinen M, Sarlomo–Rikala M. Expression of calretinin, thrombomodulin, keratin 5, and mesothelin in lung carcinomas of different types: an immunohistochemical analysis of 596 tumors in comparison with epithelioid mesotheliomas of the pleura. Am J Surg Pathol 2003;27:150–8.
12. Osborn M, Pelling N, Walker MM, et al. The value of 'mesothelium-associated' antibodies in distinguishing between metastatic renal cell carcinomas and mesotheliomas. Histopathology 2002;41:301–7.
13. Jasani B, Edwards RE, Thomas ND, et al. The use of vimentin antibodies in the diagnosis of malignant mesothelioma. Virchows Arch A Pathol Anat 1985; 406:441–8.
14. Attanoos RL, Griffin A, Gibbs AR. The use of immunohistochemistry in distinguishing reactive from neoplastic mesothelium: a novel use for desmin and comparative evaluation with epithelial membrane antigen, p53, platelet-derived

growth factor-receptor, P-glycoprotein and Bcl-2. Histopathology 2003;43: 231–8.
15. Hurlimann J. Desmin and neural marker expression in mesothelial cells and mesotheliomas. Hum Pathol 1994;25:753–7.
16. Mayall FG, Goddard H, Gibbs AR. Intermediate filament expression in mesotheliomas: leiomyoid mesotheliomas are not uncommon. Histopathology 1992;21:453–7.
17. Kung IT, Thallas V, Spencer EJ, et al. Expression of muscle actins in diffuse mesotheliomas. Hum Pathol 1995;26:565–70.
18. Doglioni C, Tos AP, Laurino L, et al. Calretinin: a novel immunocytochemical marker for mesothelioma. Am J Surg Pathol 1996;20:1037–46.
19. Tos AP, Doglioni C. Calretinin: a novel tool for diagnostic immunohistochemistry. Adv Anat Pathol 1998;5:61–6.
20. Lantuejoul S, Laverriere MH, Sturm N, et al. NCAM (neural cell adhesion molecules) expression in malignant mesotheliomas. Hum Pathol 2000;31:415–21.
21. Ordonnez NG. Application of mesothelin immunostaining in tumor diagnosis. Am J Surg Pathol 2003;27:1418–28.
22. Robinson BW, Creaney J, Lake R, et al. Mesothelin-family proteins and diagnosis of mesothelioma. Lancet 2003; 362:1612–6.
23. Rajasekaran AB. Mesothelin-family proteins: a novel diagnostic marker for malignant mesothelioma? Thorax 2004;59:143.
24. Roberts F, Harper CM, Downie I, et al. Immunohistochemical analysis still has a limited role in the diagnosis of malignant mesothelioma: a study of thirteen antibodies. Am J Clin Pathol 2001;116:253–62.
25. Roberts F, McCall AE, Burnett RA. Malignant mesothelioma: a comparison of biopsy and postmortem material by light microscopy and immunohistochemistry. J Clin Pathol 2001;54:766–70.
26. Fleury-Feith J, Kheuang L, Zeng L, et al. Human malignant mesothelial cells: variability of ultrastructural features in established and nude mice transplanted cell lines. J Pathol 1995;177:209–15.
27. Ordonez NG, Mackay B. Electron microscopy in tumor diagnosis: indications for its use in the immunohistochemical era. Hum Pathol 1998;29:1403–11.
28. Oury TD, Hammar SP, Roggli VL. Ultrastructural features of diffuse malignant mesotheliomas. Hum Pathol 1998;29:1382–92.
29. Comin CE, de Klerk NH, Henderson DW. Malignant mesothelioma: current conundrums over risk estimates and whither electron microscopy for diagnosis? Ultrastruct Pathol 1997;21:315–20.
30. Eyden BP, Banik S, Harris M. Malignant epithelial mesothelioma of the peritoneum: observations on a problem case. Ultrastruct Pathol 1996;20:337–44.
31. Corrin B, Dewar A. Adenocarcinoma simulating mesothelioma. Ultrastruct Pathol 1996;20:327–9.
32. Hammar SP, Bockus DE, Remington FL, et al. Mucin-positive epithelial mesotheliomas: a histochemical, immunohistochemical, and ultrastructural comparison with mucin-producing pulmonary adenocarcinomas. Ultrastruct Pathol 1996;20:293–325.
33. Cook DS, Attanoos RK, Jalloh SS, et al. 'Mucin positive' epithelial mesothelioma of the peritoneum: an unusual diagnostic pitfall. Histopathology 2000;17: 33–6.

34. Mayall FG, Gibbs AR. The histology and immunohistochemistry of small cell mesothelioma. Histopathology 1992;20:47–51.
35. Mayall FG, Jasani B, Gibbs AR. Immunohistochemical positivity for neuron-specific enolase and leu-7 in malignant mesotheliomas. J Pathol 1991;165:325–8.
36. Nascimento AG, Keeney GL, Fletcher CD. Deciduoid peritoneal mesothelioma: an unusual phenotype affecting young females. Am J Surg Pathol 1994; 18:439–45.
37. Shanks JH, Harris M, Banerjee SS, et al. Mesotheliomas with deciduoid morphology: a morphologic spectrum and a variant not confined to young females. Am J Surg Pathol 2000;24:285–94.
38. Butnor KJ, Burchette JL, Sporn TA, et al. The spectrum of Kit (CD117) immunoreactivity in lung and pleural tumors: a study of 96 cases using a single-source antibody with a review of the literature. Arch Pathol Lab Med 2004; 128:538–43.
39. Shia J, Erlandson RA, Klimstra DS. Deciduoid mesothelioma: a report of 5 cases and literature review. Ultrastruct Pathol 2002;26:355–63.
40. Cavazza A, Pasquinelli G, Agostini L, et al. Foamy cell mesothelioma. Histopathology 2002;41:369–71.
41. Chang HT, Yantiss RK, Nielsen GP, et al. Lipid-rich diffuse malignant mesothelioma: a case report. Hum Pathol 2000;31:876–9.
42. Ordonez NG, Mackay B. Glycogen-rich mesothelioma. Ultrastruct Pathol 1999; 23:401–6.
43. Ordonez NG, Myhre M, Mackay B. Clear cell mesothelioma. Ultrastruct Pathol 1996;20:331–6.
44. Dessy E, Falleni M, Braidotti P, et al. Unusual clear cell variant of epithelioid mesothelioma. Arch Pathol Lab Med 2001;125:1588–90.
45. Harwood TR, Gracey DR, Yokoo H. Pseudomesotheliomatous carcinoma of the lung. Am J Clin Pathol 1976;65:159–67.
46. Braganza JM, Butler EB, Fox H, et al. Ectopic production of salivary type amylase by a pseudomesotheliomatous carcinoma of the lung. Cancer 1978;41: 1522–5.
47. Dessy E, Pietra GG. Pseudomesotheliomatous carcinoma of the lung: an immunohistochemical and ultrastructural study of three cases. Cancer 1991; 68:1747–53.
48. Oka K, Otani S, Yoshimura T, et al. Mucin-negative pseudomesotheliomatous adenocarcinoma of the lung: report of three cases. Acta Oncol 1999;38:1119–21.
49. Koss M, Travis W, Moran C, et al. Pseudomesotheliomatous adenocarcinoma: a reappraisal. Semin Diagn Pathol 1992;9:117–23.
50. Attanoos RL, Gibbs AR. 'Pseudomesotheliomatous' carcinomas of the pleura: a 10-year analysis of cases from the Environmental Lung Disease Research Group, Cardiff. Histopathology 2003;43:444–52.
51. Chang YL, Lee YC, Liao WY, et al. The utility and limitation of thyroid transcription factor-1 protein in primary and metastatic pulmonary neoplasms. Lung Cancer 2004;44:149–57.
52. Zhang PJ, Livolsi VA, Brooks JJ. Malignant epithelioid vascular tumors of the pleura: report of a series and literature review. Hum Pathol 2000;31:29–34.
53. Attanoos RL, Suvarna SK, Rhead E, et al. Malignant vascular tumours of the pleura in "asbestos" workers and endothelial differentiation in malignant mesothelioma. Thorax 2000;55:860–3.

54. Essary LR, Vargas SO, Fletcher CD. Primary pleuropulmonary synovial sarcoma: reappraisal of a recently described anatomic subset. Cancer 2002;94: 459–69.
55. Attanoos RL, Galateau-Salle F, Gibbs AR, et al. Primary thymic epithelial tumour of the pleura mimicking malignant mesothelioma. Histopathology 2002; 4:42–9.
56. Corson JM. Pathology of diffuse malignant pleural mesothelioma. Semin Thorac Cardiovasc Surg 1997;9:347–55.
57. Neumann V, Gunthe S, Mulle KM, et al. Malignant mesothelioma—German mesothelioma register 1987–1999. Int Arch Occup Environ Health 2001;74: 383–95.
58. Crotty TB, Meyers JL, Katenstein AL, et al. Localized and malignant mesothelioma: a clinicopathologic and flow cytometric study. Am J Surg Pathol 1994; 18:357–63.
59. Hirano H, Takeda S, Sawabata Y, et al. Localized pleural malignant mesothelioma. Pathol Int 2003;53:616–21.
60. Allen TC, Churg A, Colby TV, et al. Localized malignant mesothelioma: clinicopathologic review of 22 cases. Mod Pathol 2004;17(Suppl 1):331A.
61. Hammar SP. Pleural diseases. In: Dail DH, Hammar SP (eds) Pulmonary pathology, 2nd edition. New York: Springer-Verlag; 1994:1463–579.
62. Battifora H, McCaughey WTE. Tumors of the serosal membranes. In: Atlas of tumor pathology, 3rd edition. Fascicle 15. Washington, DC: Armed Forces Institute of Pathology; 1995.
63. Yousem SA, Hochholzer L. Malignant mesotheliomas with osseous and cartilaginous differentiation. Arch Pathol Lab Med 1987;111:62–6.
64. Gibbs AR, Attanoos RL. Diffuse malignant mesotheliomas with heterologous differentiation.. Histopathology 2002;41(suppl 2):156–9.
65. Attanoos RL, Dojcinov S, Webb R, et al. Anti-mesothelial markers in sarcomatoid mesothelioma and other spindle cell neoplasms. Histopathology 2000;37: 224–31.
66. Oury TD, Hammar SP, Roggli VL. Ultrastructural features of diffuse malignant mesothelioma. Hum Pathol 1998;29:1382–92.
67. Travis WD, Brambilla E, Müller-Hermelink HW, et al. Pathology and genetics of tumours of the lung, pleura, thymus and heart. WHO; IARC press: Lyon 2004.
68. Wilson GE, Hasleton PS, Chattertjee A. Desmoplastic malignant mesothelioma: a review of seventeen cases. J Clin Pathol 1992;45:295–8.
69. Mangano WE, Cagle PT, Churg A, et al. The distinction from fibrous pleurisy. A histologic and immunohistochemical analysis of 31 cases including p53 immunostaining. Am J Pathol 1998;110:191–9.
70. Rapport d'activité 1998–2002 PNSM. Institut de Veille Sanitaire Hopital Saint Maurice, France; 2003.
71. Cagle PT, Brown RW, Leibowitz RM. P53 immunostaining in the differentiation of reactive processes from malignancy in pleural biopsy specimens. Hum Pathol 1994;25:443–8.
72. Mayall FG, Gibbs AR. P53 immunostaining in the distinction between benign and malignant mesothelial proliferation using formalin-fixed sections. J Pathol 1992;168:377–81.
73. Henderson DW, Attwood HD, Constance TJ, et al. Lymphohistiocytoid mesothelioma/a rare lymphomatoid variant of predominantly sarcomatoid mesothelioma. Ultrastruct Pathol 1988;12:367–84.

74. Khalidi HS, Medeiros LJ, Battifora H. Lymphohistiocytoid mesothelioma: a rare lymphomatoid variant of predominantly sarcomatoid mesothelioma. Am J Clin Pathol 2000;113:649–54.
75. Galateau-Salle F, Vignaud JM, Burke L, et al: Lymphohistiocytoïd mesothelioma: a series of 22 cases. Mod Pathol 2003;1:1402:307A.
76. Attanoos RL, Galateau-Salle F, Gibbs AR, et al. Primary thymic epithelial tumours of the pleura mimicking malignant mesothelioma. Histopathology 2002;4:42–9.

9 Differential Diagnosis: Mesothelial Proliferations

Because of the difficulty of separating benign from malignant mesothelial proliferations and malignant mesotheliomas from tumors such as carcinoma and sarcoma, it is appropriate to express levels of uncertainty in diagnostic terminology when all the data are not clear-cut. This problem often derives from inadequate specimens or conflicting results of special studies. A guiding principle is that the definitive diagnosis of malignant mesothelioma should be established based only on adequate material in the appropriate clinical context with compatible results from special studies. If there is doubt about the diagnosis, it should be reflected in the pathology report. It is better to err on the side of underdiagnosis rather than overdiagnosis. If it is a malignant mesothelioma, the tumor will ultimately declare itself. When there is uncertainty, if it is decided not to perform an additional biopsy, the patient should be followed clinically with serial radiographs to monitor for tumor progression.

Uncertainty occurs at two levels: (1) whether the lesion is benign or malignant, and (2) whether the tumor is a mesothelioma or some other type of malignancy. The following phrases are useful to employ in reports to convey various levels of uncertainty.

Atypical mesothelial proliferation
Atypical fibrous lesion of the pleura
Atypical mesothelilal proliferation, suspicious for (or consistent with/suggestive of) but not diagnostic of malignancy

Malignant epithelioid neoplasm, favor mesothelioma
Malignant epithelioid neoplasm, favor carcinoma
Malignant epithelioid neoplasm, not further classified

Malignant sarcomatoid neoplasm, favor mesothelioma
Malignant sarcomatoid neoplasm, favor sarcoma
Malignant sarcomatoid neoplasm, not further classified

For sarcomatoid neoplasms, it is unusual to encounter a pseudomesotheliomatous pattern of growth, so radiographic evidence of diffuse pleural thickening favors malignant mesothelioma. However, there are exceptions. such as synovial sarcoma, epithelioid hemangioendothelioma, and some thymic epithelial tumors that can grow in a diffuse serosal pattern.

A history of exposure to asbestos or lack thereof is important when assigning causation to a malignant mesothelioma. However, a history of exposure to asbestos should play no role in the diagnosis; the diagnosis depends on the gross and microscopic appearances and the results of special techniques, as it does with any other tumor.

Reactive Mesothelial Proliferations

The distinction of benign from malignant mesothelial proliferations can be extremely difficult, particularly because reactive serosal proliferations present a confusing array of changes involving the mesothelial surfaces, and underlying thickened and inflamed stromal tissue [1–6]. It is convenient to distinguish these processes for illustrative purposes, but the reader should remember that benign and malignant lesions may coexist.

Epithelial-type Mesothelial Proliferations Confined to a Serosal Surface

Any inflammatory stimulus in a body cavity tends to be associated with reactive changes in the surface mesothelial cells. In its simplest form, this consists of enlargement of surface cells so they take on a rounded to cuboidal configuration (Figure 9.1), a common finding in a variety of settings. Pleomorphism is more common in reactive mesothelial proliferations than typical epithelioid mesothelioma, where the nuclei can be deceptively bland. Nucleoli are often prominent in benign reactions, and mitoses may be present. In more florid proliferations, the surface cells form confluent sheets (Figure 9.2), usually without papillary cores and without lacking an underlying structure, although occasionally gland-like configurations and simple papillae are found (Figure 9.3). Formation of intracytoplasmic vacuoles (often large) is common (Figure 9.4); these vacuoles are usually negative for neutral mucin (dPAS stain), although they may stain with mucicarmine, a nonspecific finding in this setting. This finding can be helpful if the question of metastatic adenocarcinoma arises. Necrosis of surface aggregates of mesothelial cells may be seen during infectious processes, especially tuberculosis, and rarely with other benign conditions. The finding of necrosis, especially in the absence of acute inflammation, always raises the question of malignancy.

Experience has shown that invasion of the stroma is the most reliable guide to the diagnosis of malignancy in mesothelial proliferations (Figure 9.5). When a small biopsy appears to be solid tumor from one end to the other, one is usually on safe ground in concluding that the lesion is

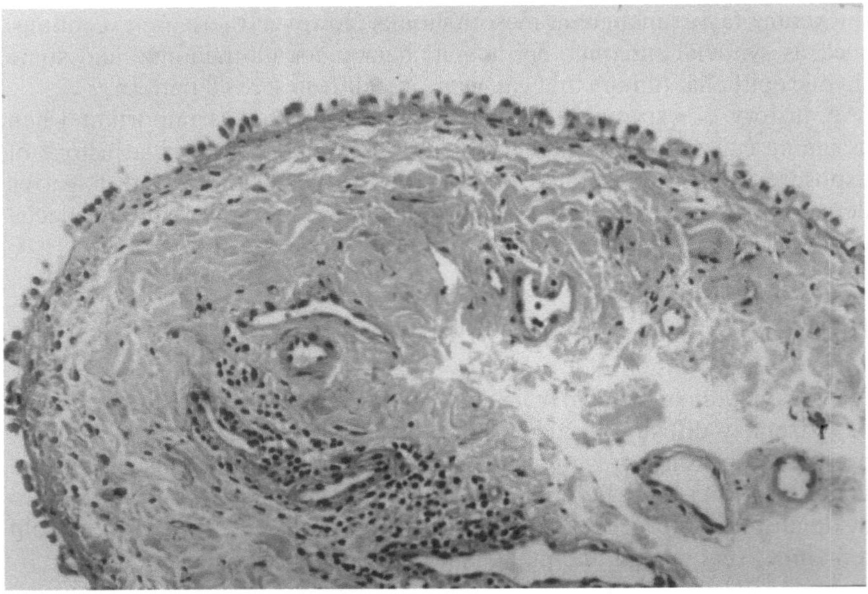

Figure 9.1. Hyperplasia of surface mesothelial cells, which are cuboidal in appearance with areas of separation.

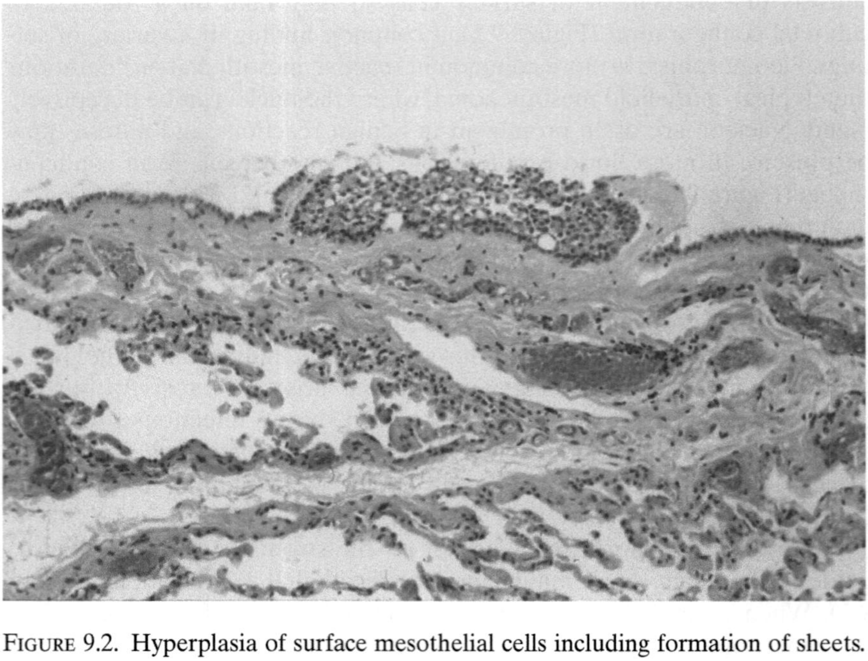

Figure 9.2. Hyperplasia of surface mesothelial cells including formation of sheets.

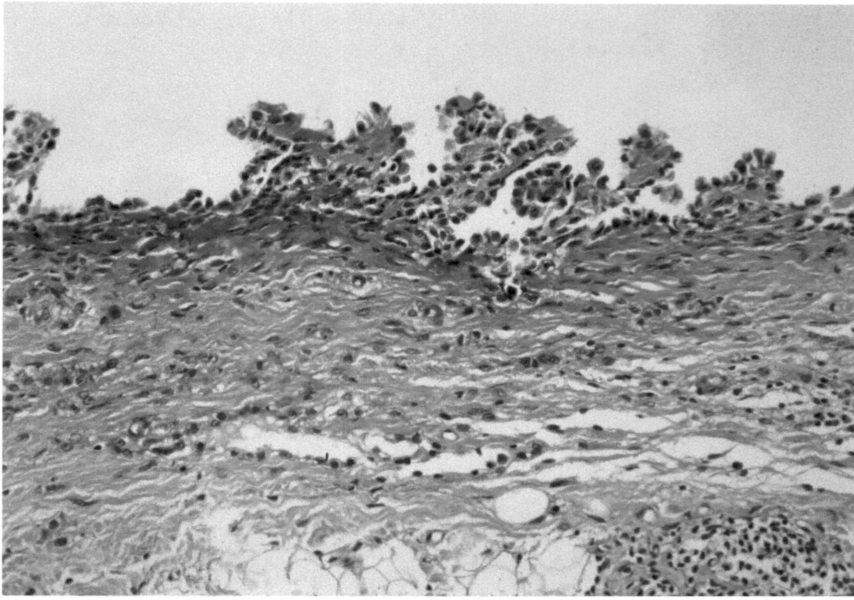

FIGURE 9.3. Papillary formation in atypical mesothelial proliferation.

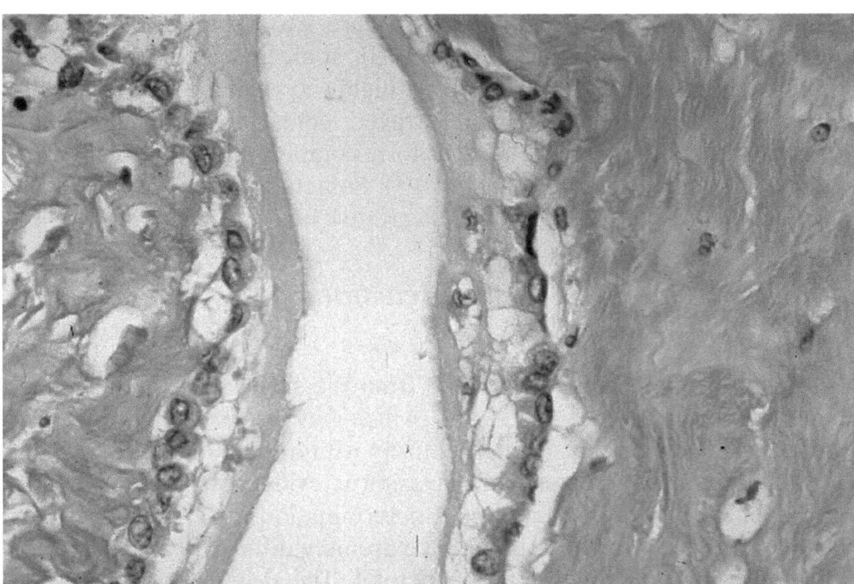

FIGURE 9.4. Mesothelial proliferation with vacuolation.

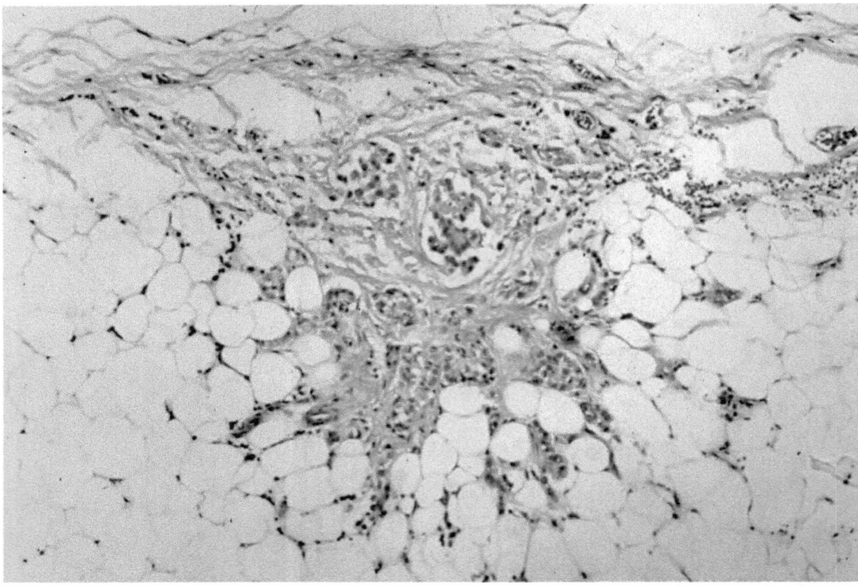

FIGURE 9.5. True invasion from epithelioid mesothelioma.

malignant. When a surface proliferation shows features suggestive of malignancy but without invasion, we propose that it be termed "atypical mesothelial proliferation" and that additional biopsies be suggested for cases clinically suspicious for mesothelioma (Figure 9.6). Atypical mesothelial hyperplasia can take a variety of forms. In some instances, the process appears large; and, cytologically, there are highly atypical single cells, usually cuboidal and occasionally columnar, arrayed along a mesothelial surface. In other instances, the mesothelial cells form complex patterns, usually with papillary inflammatory cores (Figure 9.7). Sometimes such proliferations induce their own stroma, a sign that is suggestive of malignancy (Figure 9.6).

Epithelioid-type Mesothelial Reactions in a Thickened Serous Membrane

Mesothelial proliferations may extend from the surface into a thickened, inflamed, or fibrotic serous membrane (which may also have all those characteristics), or they may be located entirely within the membrane. A good rule of thumb is that true stromal invasion is evidence of malignancy in mesothelial proliferations, although determination of invasion versus entrapment of mesothelial cells can be extremely difficult (Figure 9.5).

The following guidelines may be helpful. The distribution of epithelioid mesothelial cells (zonation) in a thickened serosal membrane is an extremely helpful guide for distinguishing benign from maligant processes.

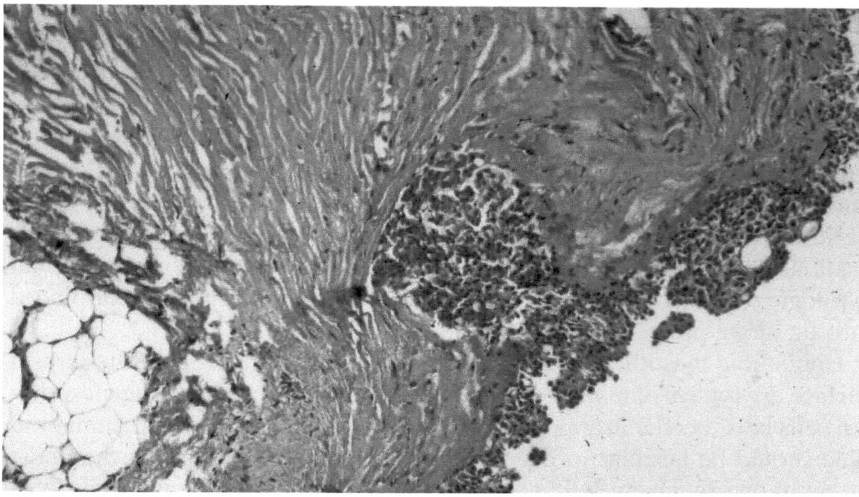

FIGURE 9.6. Vacuolated mesothelial proliferation appearing to form its own stroma. It is suspicious for malignancy.

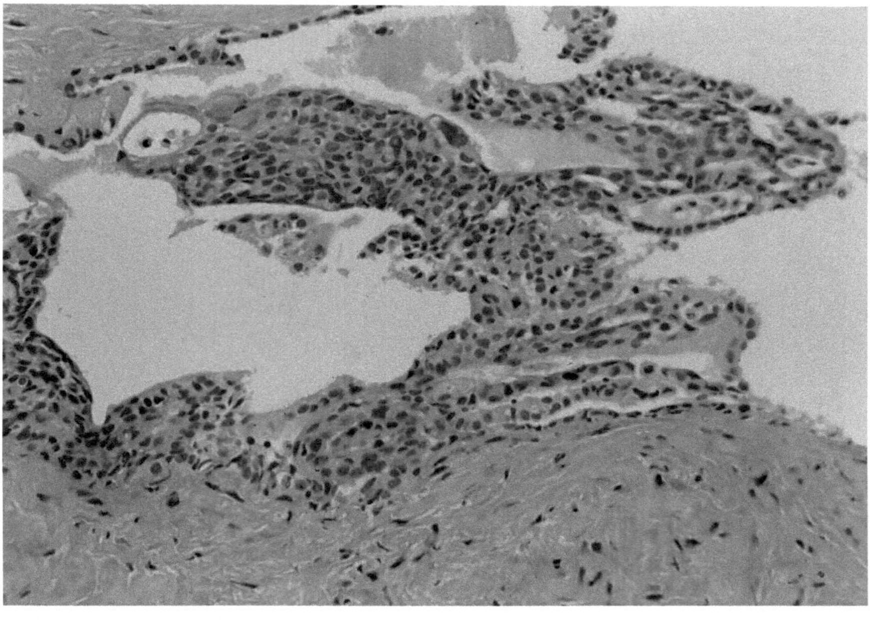

FIGURE 9.7. Complex atypical mesothelial proliferation.

In the parietal pleura, an epithelioid mesothelial proliferation that infiltrates fat or chest wall muscle is always malignant. An epithelioid mesothelial proliferation that extends across the full width of a thickened serosal membrane (e.g., from the pleural cavity to the fat) is usually malignant. This is true of epithelioid proliferations that are predominantly distributed toward the chest wall. The same comments apply to the pericardial cavity and to the peritoneal cavities. Orientation may be difficult to discern in the peritoneal cavity, but benign processes should not invade fat. Such proliferations can be deceptively bland, and distribution is more helpful than cytologic detail. Rarely, benign epithelioid proliferations may be displaced into fat along previous biopsy/needle tracts.

Epithelioid mesothelial cells located immediately underneath the serosal surface are typical of many benign reactions in which proliferating mesothelial cells have been entrapped owing to a current or previous inflammation. One should be hesitant to diagnose malignant mesothelioma in the midst of acute or organizing inflammation. Other clues to the benign nature of the process are the presence of only one or a few glands in the serous membrane. Glands or single cells forming linear arrays parallel to the serosal surface also favor benignity (Figure 9.8). This phenomenon represents layering and organization of an inflammatory exudate on a preexisting mesothelial surface and is particularly common around uterine adnexae. Fibrin may be entrapped with mesothelial cells in a benign process, but this situation also may be seen with mesothelioma.

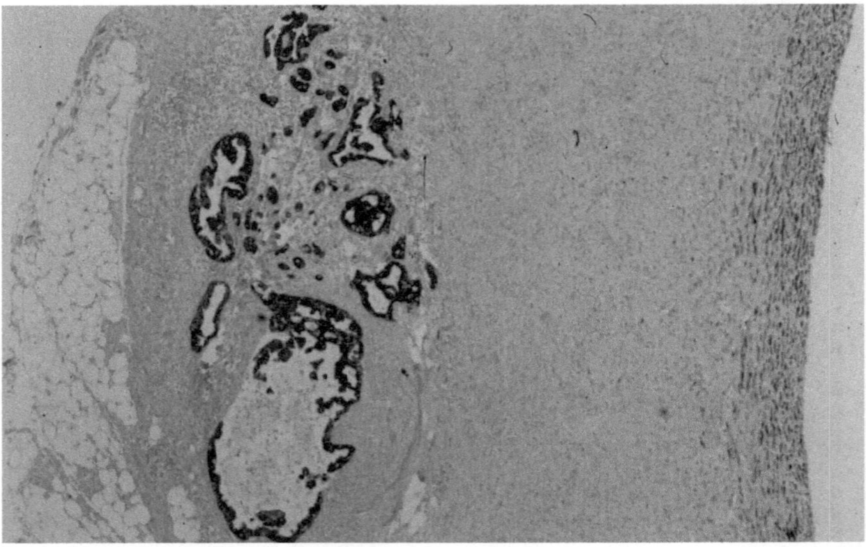

FIGURE 9.8. Sequestrated mesothelial proliferation, which could be mistaken for malignancy.

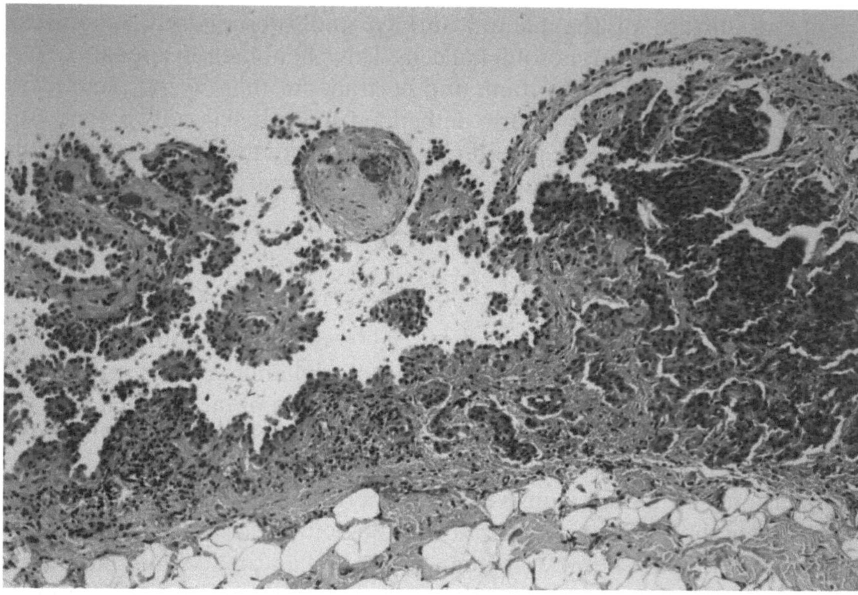

FIGURE 9.9. Complex mesothelial proliferation, showing superficial invasion indicating malignancy.

Benign epithelioid mesothelial cell proliferations typically do not show full-thickness extension through a serosal membrane. An abrupt, often linear, cutoff of proliferating mesothelial cells at a shallow depth from the surface favors a benign reaction. In the peritoneal cavity, benign mesothelial cells may become trapped between lobules of fat, where they form linear arrays but do not infiltrate the fat itself. Malignant mesotheliomas may, on occasion, also show a predominantly subserosal distribution. Clues to malignancy are complex glands, typically branching (Figure 9.6) and often forming a classic tubulopapillary pattern (Figure 9.9). Sometimes one portion of a biopsy specimen shows a subserosal proliferation that is suspicious but not diagnostic of mesothelioma, whereas other pieces or deeper sections demonstrate clearly invasive tumor. Equivocal cases should be labeled "atypical mesothelial proliferation," with more tissue requested.

Sequestration of Mesothelial Cells (Pseudoinvasion)

Reactive mesothelial hyperplasias may be accompanied by low-grade cytoarchitectural atypia. In addition, serosal inflammatory disorders may produce sequestration of mesothelial cells in the submesothelial connective tissue. With benign inflammatory processes, a layer of fibrinous exudate covers the surface of the pleural surface and subsequently organizes, leading to entrapment of mesothelial cells. This phenomenon appears to be more common in the pericardium and peritoneum than in the pleura. In both the pericardium and pleura, embedded mesothelial cells extend no deeper than the submesothelial fibrous layer, so extension into subpleural adipose tissue or deeper structures such as chest wall striated muscle is a strong indicator of malignancy.

Inclusions of Mesothelial Cells in Lymph Nodes

Rarely, lymph node metastases are the presenting manifestation of malignant mesothelioma. Conversely, chronic inflammatory disorders of serosal membranes are associated with translocation of mesothelial cells to regional lymph nodes. In some benign mesothelial cell inclusions, the cells are restricted to the subcapsular sinus (Figure 9.10), whereas in other cases the inclusions are more extensive, with penetration into the deeper nodal tissue; under these circumstances, no histologic criteria have been formulated to discriminate between benign inclusions and metastatic mesothelioma [7, 8]. Therefore a diagnostic biopsy of the corresponding serosal membrane or radiologic evidence supportive of an underlying mesothelioma is mandatory before a diagnosis of metastatic mesothelioma can be established.

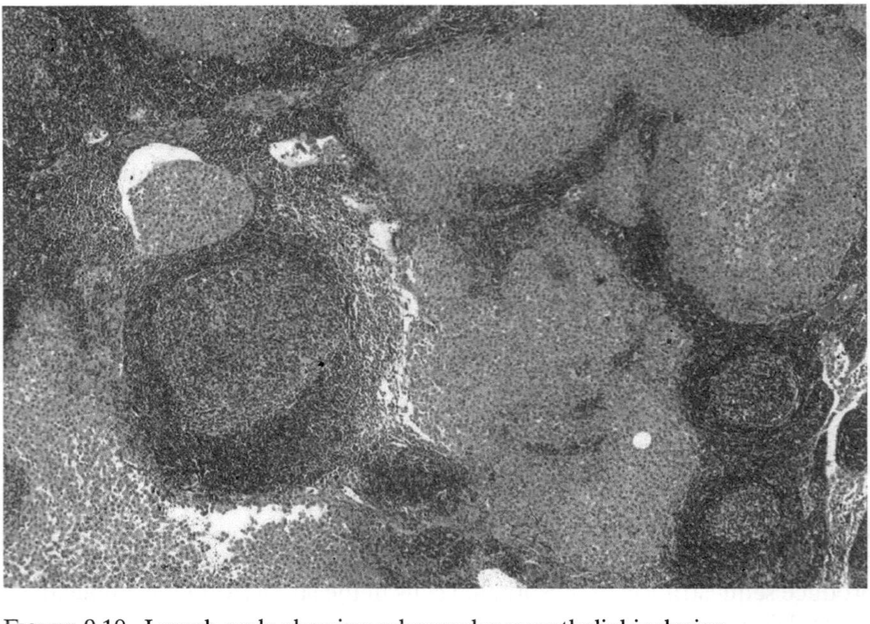

FIGURE 9.10. Lymph node showing subcapsular mesothelial inclusion.

Fibrous Pleurisy

Sarcomatoid and desmoplastic mesotheliomas are discussed above, but benign reactions in which the proliferating mesothelial cells are entirely or mostly spindled also occur and are termed "fibrous pleurisy" (other terms are fibrous pleuritis, fibrosing pleuritis, organizing pleurisy). Equivalent reactions may be seen in other serosal membranes and can be descriptively termed fibrosing peritonitis and fibrosing pericarditis.

Like benign epithelial proliferations, fibrous pleurisy is associated with distinct zonation, with greater cellularity immediately underneath the surface layer and progressive loss of cellularity and increasing stromal fibrosis toward the chest wall (Figures 9.11 and 9.12). Plaque may be subsumed by tumor and cause problems of interpretation. By contrast, desmoplastic and sarcomatoid mesotheliomas usually have no zonation and are often homogeneously distributed through a thickened serosal membrane or are more prominent toward the chest wall.

The cells immediately under the surface layer of the serosa in fibrous pleurisy are cytologically atypical and spindled, similar to those at the base of active peptic ulcers in the gastrointestinal tract. They are usually admixed with fibrin but do not extend deep into the thickened pleura. These cells have the morphologic features of myofibroblasts. As one moves further

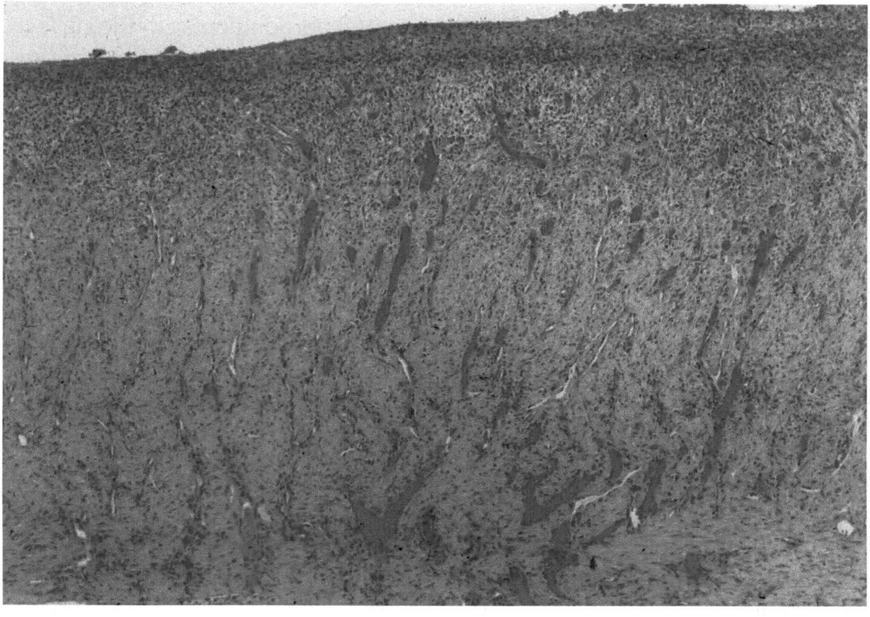

FIGURE 9.11. Long capillaries oriented perpendicular to the pleural surface are a sign of benign fibrous pleurisy.

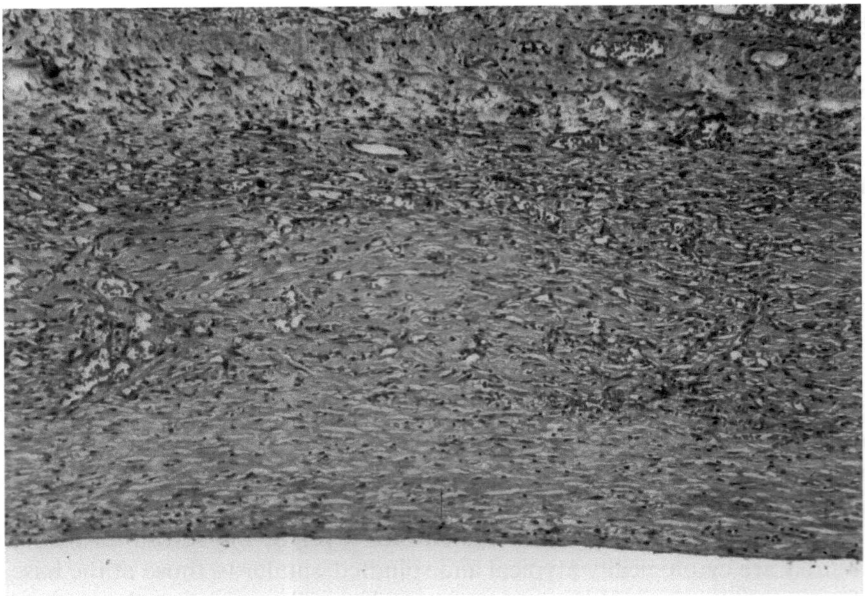

FIGURE 9.12. Systemic lupus erythematosus, showing fibrinous chronic inflammation of the pleura.

away from the surface, long capillaries oriented perpendicular to the surface (Figure 9.11) may be found. Their presence is helpful because they are typically not a feature of sarcomatoid or desmoplastic mesotheliomas. Usually the spindle cells in fibrous pleurisy do not extend into the fat; but such extension and even the production of fibrous tissue surrounding chest wall muscle may be seen with a fibrothorax and with prior surgery (Figure 9.13). As noted above, both benign and malignant spindle cell mesothelial proliferations are usually keratin-positive. Insinuation of keratin-positive cells between fat cells is a characteristic feature of desmoplastic or sarcomatoid mesotheliomas.

Plaques

Because most mesotheliomas are caused by asbestos, the parietal pleura often also shows accompanying hyaline pleural plaques, which are markers of asbestos exposure but not of asbestosis. Plaques do not predispose to the development of malignancy but may be encountered in the vicinity of a mesothelioma. They are observed most frequently on the diaphragmatic parietal pleura (Figure 9.14) and the lateral chest wall, usually in the distribution of the ribs. Plaques are rarely seen on the visceral pleura or

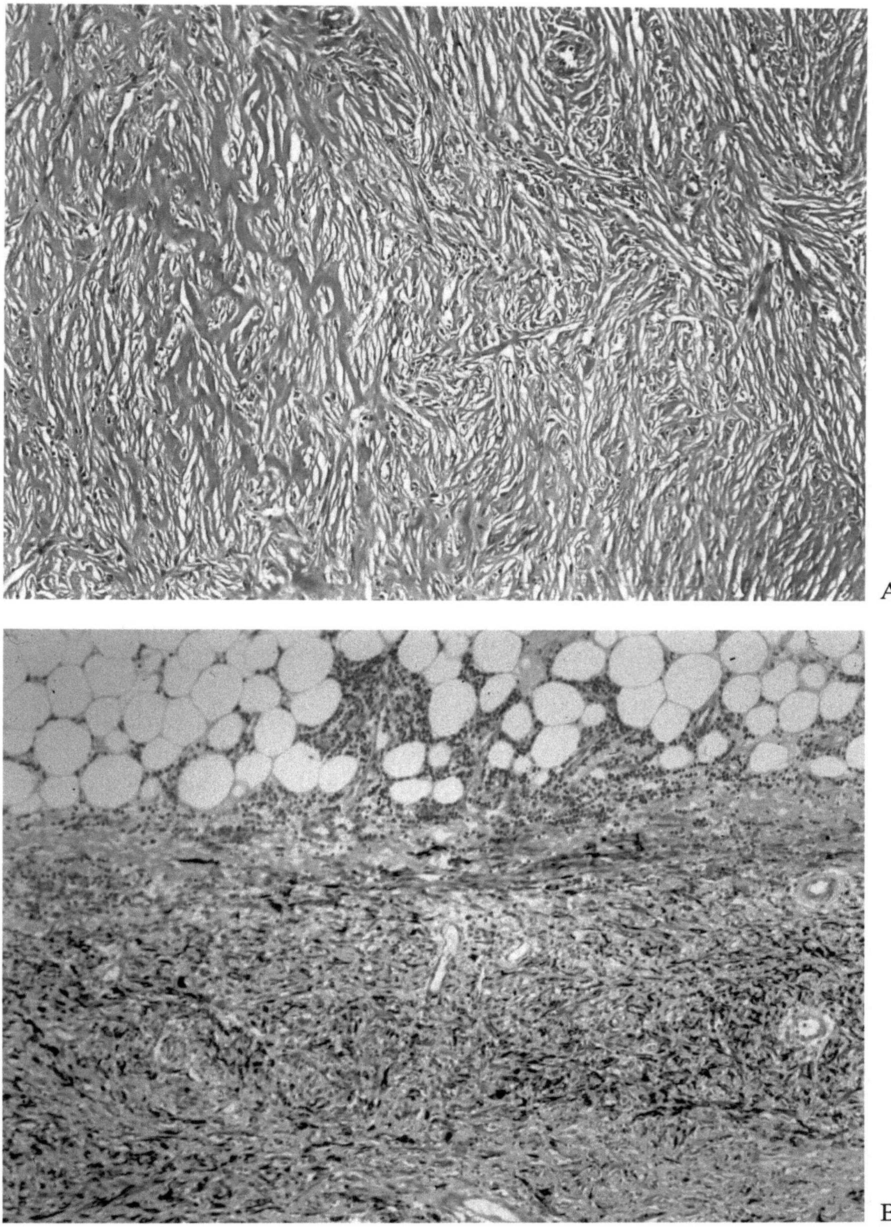

FIGURE 9.13. A. Highly cellular asbestos-related pleural fibrosis. B. Same case. showing the absence of invasion of adipose tissue by reactive stromal cells. (Cytokeratin immunostaining)

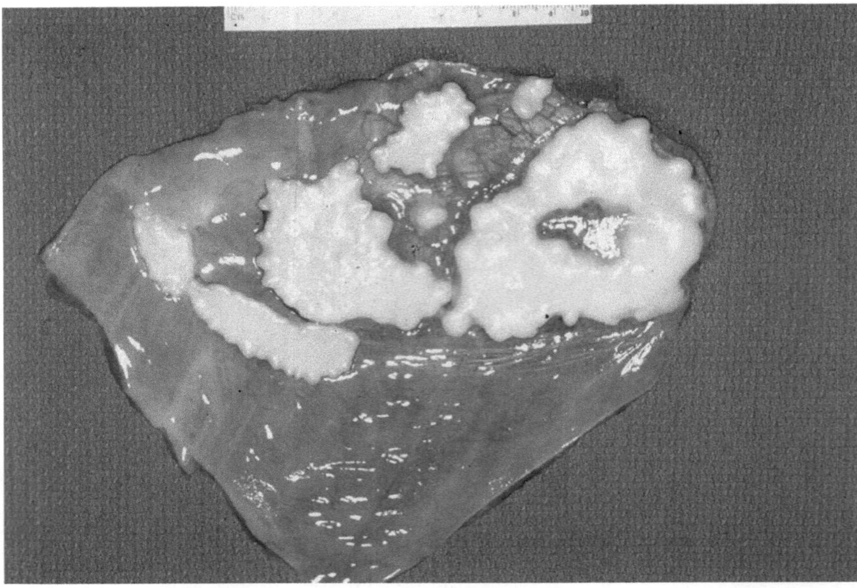

FIGURE 9.14. Pearly gray nodular diaphragmatic parietal pleural plaques.

visceral pericardium. Plaques identical to those seen on the parietal pleura have been observed on the peritoneal surface, most frequently on the spleen or liver. Grossly, they are white or yellow lesions that are histologically composed of a basket-weave pattern of acellular collagen sharply demarcated from the underlying tissue. They express pancytokeratin and should not be confused with desmoplastic mesothelioma.

The prevalence of plaques in the general population and in association with malignant mesothelioma varies considerably according to the population studied and the method of detection. For example, Roggli et al. [9], reported that 71% of mesotheliomas were associated with plaques in U.S. men, and Bianchi et al. reported almost 90% in Italian men and 70% in women based on autopsy results[10].

Peritoneal Fibrosis/Sclerosing Fibrosis

Peritoneal fibrosis/sclerosing fibrosis are reactive processes characterized by peritoneal fibrosis that may encase the bowel, causing severe obstruction. They may be misdiagnosed as desmoplastic malignant mesothelioma, particularly in a closed biopsy specimen. Multipotential subserosal cells are well known for presenting pancytokeratin or calretinin positivity in both benign and malignant mesothelial lesions. In this situation, invasion of adipose tissue between adipocytes is the clue to the correct diagnosis. Peritonal fibrosis usually occurs in the setting of abdominal operations, whereas sclerosing peritonitis may be idiopathic or secondary to chronic ambulatory peritoneal dialysis. It also may occur in association with fibrothecoma of the ovary and may mimic a malignant process [11].

Fibrous Periorchitis

Fibrous periorchitis is a diffuse or localized reactive process involving the tunica vaginalis, the epididymis, and the spermatic cord. It has been described under various names such as nodular fibrous periorchitis, nodular pseudotumor, fibrous mesothelioma, and proliferative funiculitis. It is thought to be a reactive process characterized by diffuse thickening or a localized process made of multiple fibrous nodules 0.2 to 10.0 cm in diameter. Histologically, it is composed of spindle cells and hyalinized collagen. An inflammatory component may be prominent. These lesions should be differentiated from desmoplastic malignant mesothelioma and lymphohistiocytoid mesothelioma, which have not been described to our knowledge at this site. It should also be differentiated from sarcomas, which are generally more atypical and cellular [12].

Immunohistochemical Findings in Reactive Versus Neoplastic Processes

Positive staining with broad-spectrum anti-keratin is not a feature specific for malignancy but can be seen in every active mesothelial proliferation, benign or malignant, epithelioid or spindled. Keratin staining is helpful, however, in showing the distribution of mesothelial cells in serosal membranes. This is especially true for showing linear arrays (favoring a benign process) and subtle penetration into fat or other structures (suggesting malignancy).

Published studies have reported that neoplastic epithelioid mesothelial cells show cell membrane staining (often thick) for epithelial membrane antigen (EMA) (Figure 9.15) and human milk fat globule protein-2 (HMFG-2), whereas reactive atypical epithelial mesothelial cells are usually nonreactive. Similarly, neoplastic mesothelial cells more frequently express p53 gene product than do reactive mesothelial cells. Caution is urged when using these reactions to establish a diagnosis because reactive epithelial mesothelial cells may express EMA, HMFG-2, and p53, and neoplastic epithelial mesothelial cells may show no reactivity [13].

Desmin also appears to be preferentially expressed in reactive mesothelium. The complementary use of EMA and desmin markers may be of pratical value in ascertaining the nature of mesothelial proliferations [14–16]. Immunohistochemical detection of mutated *p53* oncoprotein is more controversial. All these markers are useful but not definitively diagnostic, and they require more formal evaluation in the future.

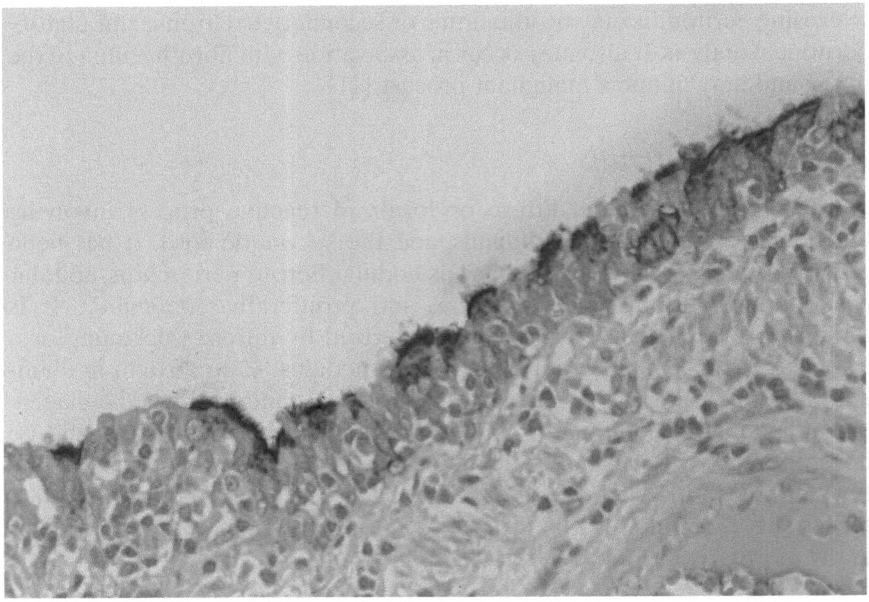

FIGURE 9.15. Mesothelial proliferation, showing focal membranous immunostaining for epithelial membrane antigen (EMA).

References

1. Bolen JW, Hammar SP, McNutt MA. Reactive and neoplastic serosal tissue: a light-microscopic, ultrastructural, and immunocytochemical study. Am J Surg Pathol 1986;10:34–47.
2. Bolen JW, Hammar SP, McNutt MA. Serosal tissue: reactive tissue as a model for understanding mesotheliomas. Ultrastruct Pathol 1987;11:251–62.
3. Whitaker D, Manning LS, Robinson BWS, et al. The pathology of the mesothelium. In: Henderson DW, Shilkin KB, Langlois SLP, et al (eds) Malignant mesothelioma. New York: Hemisphere; 1991:25–68.
4. Henderson DW, Shilkin KB, Whitaker D. Reactive mesothelial hyperplasia versus mesothelioma, including mesothelioma in situ. Am J Clin Pathol 1998; 110:397–404.
5. Churg A, Colby TV, Cagle P, et al. The separation of benign and malignant mesothelial cell proliferations. Am J Surg Pathol 2000;24:1183–2000.
6. Galateau-Salle F, Cagle P. Non malignant versus malignant proliferations on pleural biopsy: In: Cagle P (ed) Diagnostic pulmonary pathology. New York: Marcel Dekker; 2000.
7. Brooks JSJ, Livolsi V, Pietra GG. Mesothelial cell inclusions in mediastinal lymph nodes mimicking metastatic carcinoma. Am J Clin Pathol 1990;93:741–8.
8. Parkash V, Vidwans M, Carter D. Benign mesothelial cells in mediastinal lymph nodes. Am J Surg Pathol 1999;23:1264–9.

9. Roggli VL, Sharm A, Butnor KJ, et al. Malignant mesothelioma and occupational exposure to asbestos: a clinicopathological correlation of 1445 cases. Ultrastruct Pathol 2002;26:55–65.
10. Bianchi C, Brollo A, Ramani L, et al. Pleural plaques as risk indicators for malignant pleural mesothelioma: a necropsy based study. Am J Ind Med 1997; 32:445–9.
11. Clement PB, Young RH, Hanna W, et al. Sclerosing peritonitis associated with luteinized thecomas of the ovary; a clinicopathological analysis of six cases. Am J Surg Pathol 1994;18:1–13.
12. Jones MA, Young RH, Scully RE. Benign fibromatous tumors of the testis and the paratesticular region: a report of 9 cases with proposed classification of fibromatous tumors and tumor-like lesions. Am J Surg Pathol 1997;21:296–305.
13. Cury PM, Butcher DN, Corrin B, et al. The use of histological and immunohistochemical markers to distinguish pleural mesothelioma and in situ mesothelioma from reactive mesothelial hyperplasia and reactive pleural fibrosis. J Pathol 1999;189:251–7.
14. Attanoos RL, Griffin A, Gibbs AR. The use of immunohistochemistry in distinguishing reactive from neoplastic mesothelium: a novel use for desmin and comparative evaluation with epithelial membrane antigen, p53, platelet-derived growth factor-receptor, P-glycoprotein and Bcl-2. Histopathology 2003;43: 231–8.
15. Hurlimann J. Desmin and neural marker expression in mesothelial cells and mesotheliomas. Hum Pathol 1994;25:753–7.
16. Afify AM, Al-Khafaji BM, Paulino AF, et al. Diagnostic use of muscle markers in the cytologic evaluation of serous fluids. Appl Immunohistochem Mol Morphol 2002;10:178–82.

10 Differential Diagnosis: Other Mesothelial Lesions

Adenomatoid Tumors

Characteristically, adenomatoid tumors are benign proliferations of mesothelial cells that occur most frequently in the testis/epididymis and in the cornua of the uterus. Rarely, the tumor has been described in the pleura (Figure 10.1) [1]. Adenomatoid tumors appear infiltrative and can be confused with other types of neoplasms.

Adenomatoid tumors are usually clinically silent, occurring as genital tract tumors in both males and females. They are most often discovered incidentally as a minute polypoid, pedunculated, or sessile nodule on surgical specimens. They have no relation to asbestos exposure. Microscopically, these tumors of the pleura display a proliferation of large epithelioid cells arranged in trabeculae, with gland-like spaces and containing intracytoplasmic vacuoles (Figure 10.2). The cells are devoid of atypia. Lymphoid follicles are frequently seen at the edge of the polypoid pedicle. Immunohistochemically, the cells are cytokeratin- and calretinin-positive and show no immunostaining for carcinoma markers. The lesion is considered benign, but some cases with malignant behavior have been described in the genital tract. A useful feature for differentiating adenomatoid pleural tumor from the signet ring and adenoid cystic variants of malignant mesothelioma is that the former lesion is minute and measures less than 5 mm. These lesions may also be misinterpreted as epithelioid hemangioendotheliomas, but they are CD31- and CD34-positive and are usually cytokeratin-negative.

The diagnosis of benign adenomatoid tumor of the pleura should be restricted to rare cases fulfilling the following criteria: (1) the nodule is small (<5 mm) and is an incidental finding at operation performed for other reasons; (2) symptoms are restricted to the disorder for which the operative procedure was carried out, and there is no effusion attributable to the pleural nodule; and (3) the appearances throughout the nodule are characteristic of an adenomatoid tumor, with no histologic features characteristic of malignant mesothelioma (e.g., tubulopapillary structures at the surface of the pleura or a sarcomatoid component).

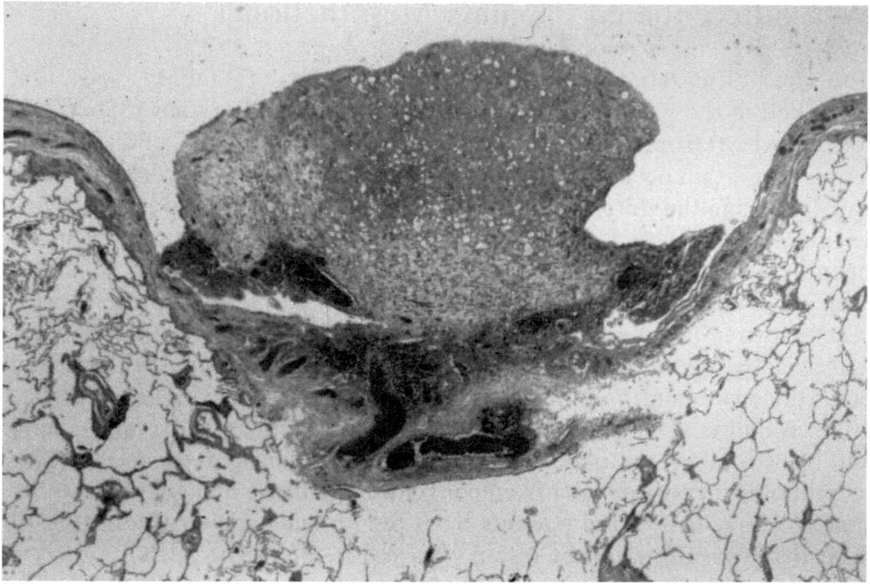

FIGURE 10.1. Low power view of pleural adenomatoid tumor.

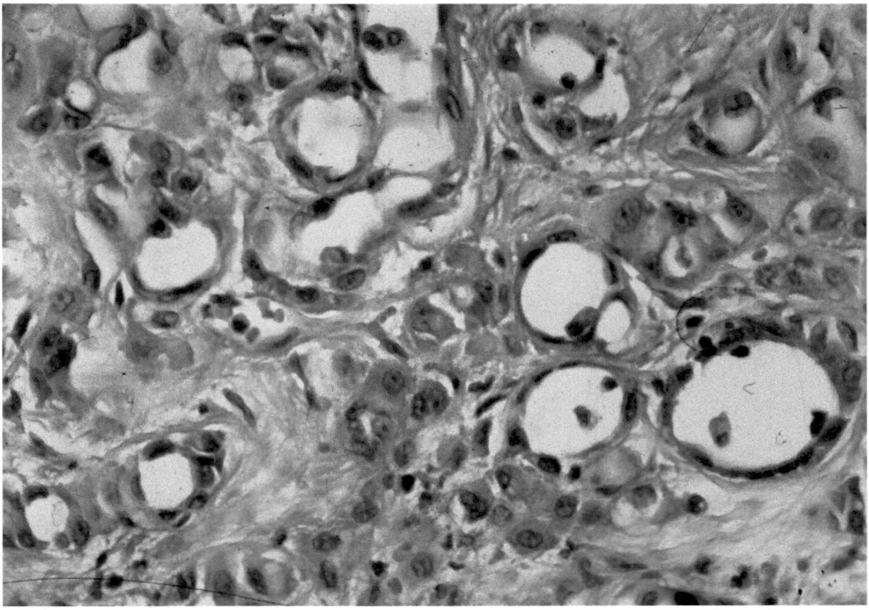

FIGURE 10.2. High power view of pleural adenomatoid tumor.

Well-differentiated Papillary Mesothelioma

The well-differentiated papillary mesothelioma (WDPM) was first described in the peritoneum by Foyle et al. in 1981 [2]. Other reports followed in 1990 from Daya and McCaughey [3] and Ascensio et al. [4]. It is a rare tumor that occurs predominantly in the peritoneum of young women, usually during the third decade. It has also been encountered in the tunica vaginalis of the testis [5, 6] as well as in the female genital tract [7]. It has been described in the pleura [8–10], where it is even more rare. It affects men and women equally, with a mean age of 60 years, and it presents with recurrent free-flowing unilateral pleural effusion. Histologically, it is characterized by superficial spreading of stout papillary formations with myxoid cores lined by bland, flattened cells with or without limited invasion (Figure 10.3). WDPMs are associated with an indolent clinical course and a long survival (from 3 years to more than 10 years). It is considered a specific clinicopathologic entity distinct from conventional diffuse malignant mesothelioma. Nearly half of the patients from the French series had a history of asbestos exposure when the lesion occurred in the pleura [10].

Macroscopically WDPM presents in the pleura as multiple small, pinpoint nodules usually less than 1 cm. Localized disease may appear as a solitary nodule often with a stalk attached to the mesothelial surface.

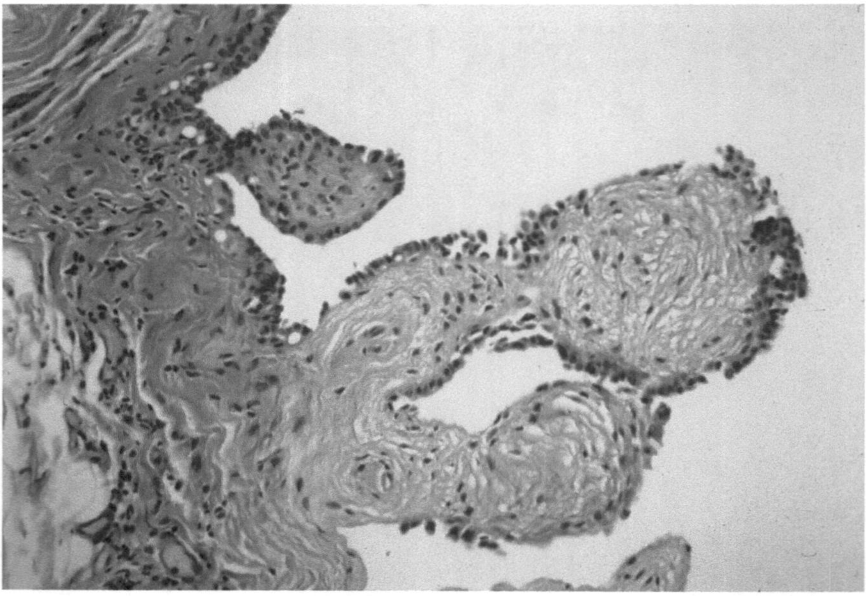

FIGURE 10.3. Visceral pleura: well-differentiated papillary mesothelioma with surface papillary formation.

Histologically, the proliferation expands from the serosal surface of the peritoneum or the pleura, and there is a well developed papillary pattern (Figure 10.4). WDMPs are characterized by a bland cytology. Moreover, invasion is absent or extremely limited, as it is mostly a superficial process.

In the pleura, the major difficulty for the differential diagnosis is with atypical mesothelial hyperplasia in a recurrent pleural effusion secondary to a previous cardiovascular inflammatory, immune, or toxic disease. According to Galateau-Salle et al. [10], immunohistochemical stains demonstrated 100% membranous staining for epithelial membrane antigen (EMA) (Figure 10.5). The usefulness of p53 in differentiating WDPMs from reactive atypical hyperplasia has not been well established.

In the peritoneum, WDPM is usually an incidental finding at surgery and is not related to prior asbestos exposure [11]. The tumor pursues a benign or indolent course, or when multiple lesions are present they can give rise to ascites. Some cases have been reported with persistent or progressive disease [11]. The main differential diagnosis includes focal mesothelial reactive hyperplasia and the spectrum of serous peritoneal tumors, including borderline serous tumor of the peritoneum, as well as serous papillary carcinoma of the ovary and diffuse malignant epithelioid mesothelioma [7, 12–14].

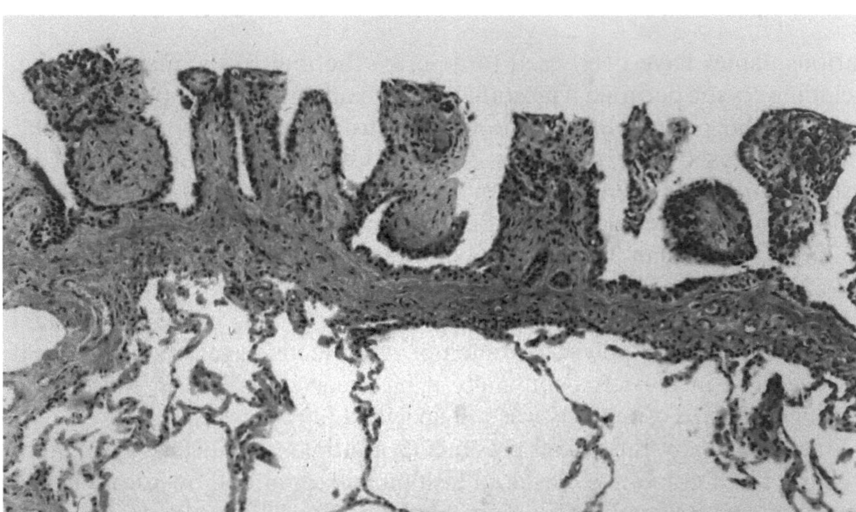

FIGURE 10.4. Well-differentiated papillary mesothelioma with uniform papillae containing myxoid fibrous cores lined by a single layer of bland mesothelial cells.

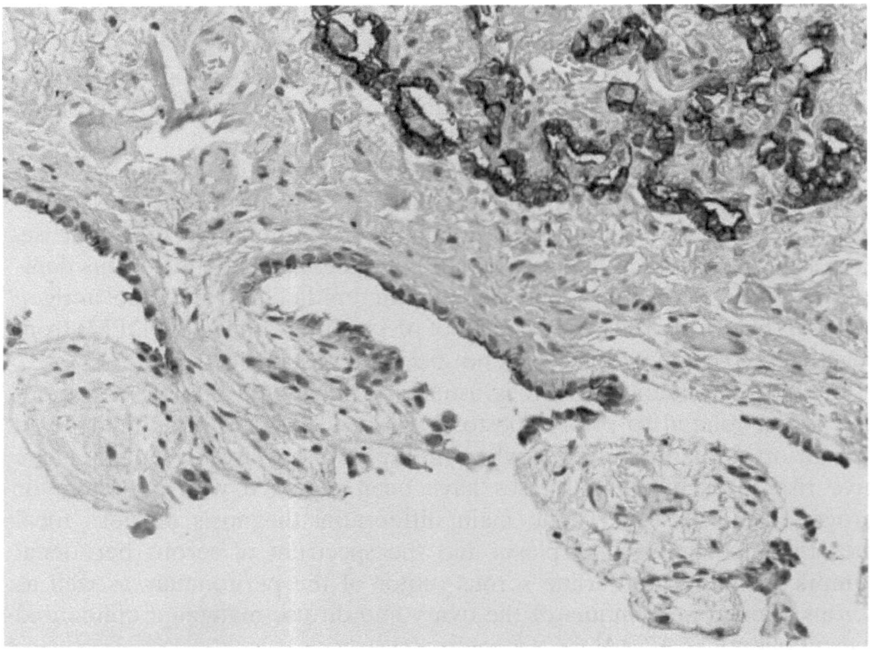

FIGURE 10.5. Well-differentiated papillary mesothelioma with uniform papillae showing focal membranous epithelial membrane antigen immunostaining.

Multicystic Mesothelioma

Various names have been used to describe the multicystic mesothelioma, including "cystic peritoneal mesothelioma," "inflammatory or postoperative cysts" of the peritoneum, "peritoneal inclusion cysts," and "multilocular peritoneal cysts." The diagnosis of multicystic mesothelioma should be restricted to cases where the tumor is completely cystic, with the cysts large enough to be detected by naked-eye examination. They may be as large as 20cm. More than 100 cases have been documented in the literature [15–22].

Multicystic mesothelioma is a rare disease, occurring in the peritoneum and especially in the pelvis in women of reproductive age. In some cases it has occurred in men. Exceptionally it has been described in the pleura, although the size of the cyts was not specified [20].

Macroscopically, this lesion presents as multiple translucents cysts often organized in a grape-like clustered fashion and separated by fibrous septa. The cysts contain a gelatinous, mucinous fluid [21–22].

Microscopically, multicystic mesotheliomas (multicystic peritoneal cysts) are lined by a single layer of flattened or hobnail-shaped epithelioid cells with no or mild cellular atypia (Figure 10.6). The cyst walls are composed

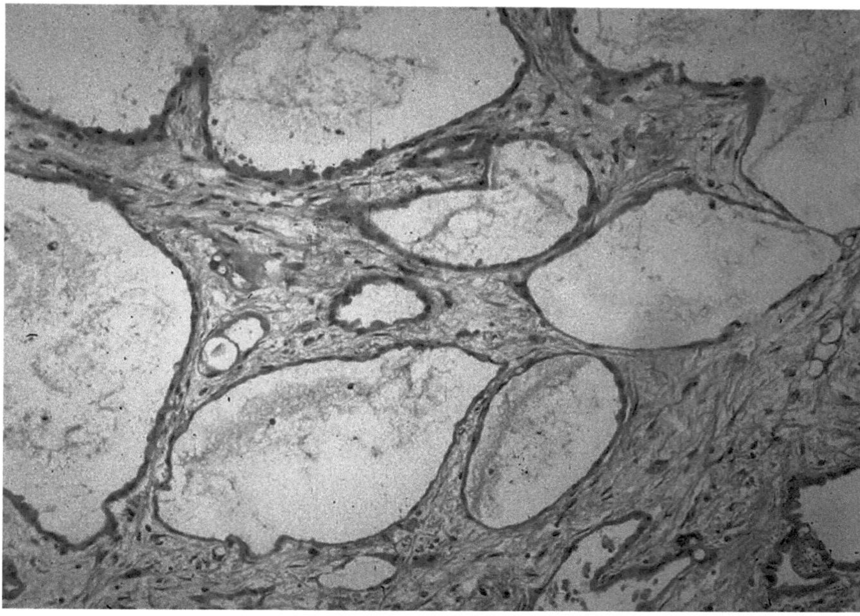

FIGURE 10.6. Multicystic mesothelioma.

of dense fibrovascular connective tissue scattered with a few inflammatory cells (Figure 10.7). Neoplastic infiltration of the adjacent fibrous tissue is absent. Adenomatoid tumors have been associated in rare cases [15, 17, 21, 23]. The mesothelial cells lining the cysts show positive immunostaining for AE1/AE3, CK5/6, CK7, HBME-1, and calretinin; EMA expression is variable, and endothelial markers are negative.

There is some controversy regarding the nature of this lesion. Some multicystic mesotheliomas appear to be reactive as they develop in association with prior pelvic surgery, pelvic inflammatory disease, or endometriosis. Others, presenting with repeated recurrences, are probably neoplastic. The latter should be considered low grade malignant bona fide multicystic mesotheliomas, whereas the former are better interpreted as peritoneal or multilocular peritoneal reactive cysts.

Mesotheliomas are rare during childhood. When they do appear, they may have a multicystic appearance and unpredictable behavior, requiring individual treatment strategies [23, 24]. Multicystic mesothelioma does not appear to be related to asbestos exposure.

The major differential diagnosis includes a conventional epithelioid mesothelioma with an adenomatoid appearance; if there is an associated invasive component, the lesions should be regarded as a diffuse malignant mesothelioma. Additional differential diagnoses include cystic lymphangioma [25] and endosalpingiosis [26]. The former stains positively for CD31,

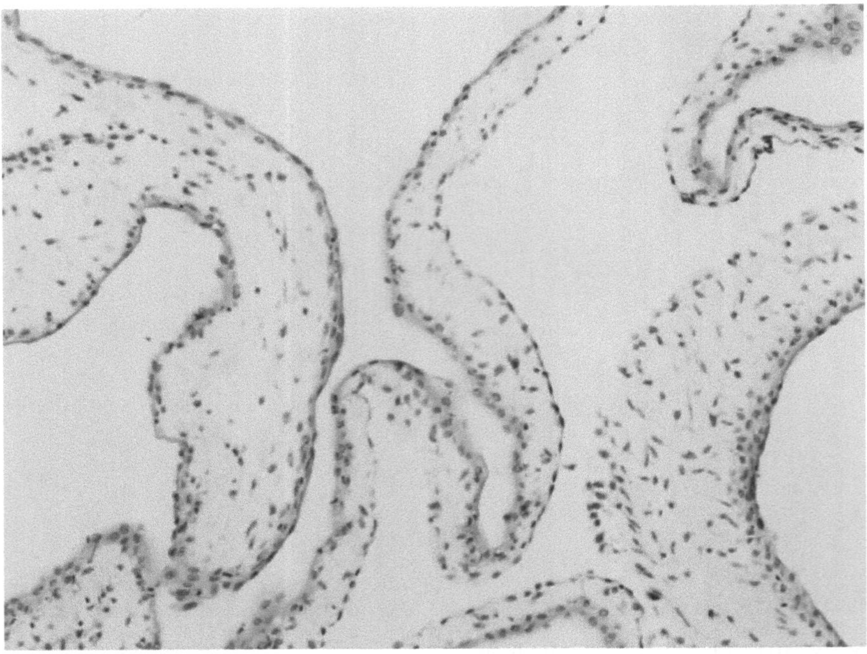

FIGURE 10.7. Peritoneal cysts are lined by a single layer of flat cuboidal cells with benign nuclear features.

factor VIIII-related antigen, and vimentin and does not express mesothelial markers.

References

1. Kaplan MA, Tazelaar HD, Hayashi T, et al. Adenomatoid tumor of the pleura. Am J Surg Pathol 1995;19:659–65.
2. Foyle A, Al-Jabi M, McCaughey WTE. Papillary peritoneal tumors in women. Am J Surg Pathol 1981;5:241–9.
3. Daya D, McCaughey WTE. Well differentiated papillary mesothelioma of the peritoneum: a clinicopathologic study of 22 cases. Cancer 1990;65:292–6.
4. Asensio JA, Goldblatt P, Thomford NR. Primary malignant peritoneal mesothelioma: a report of seven cases and a review of the literature. Arch Surg 1990; 25:1477–81.
5. Coue O, Depinieux G, Lamy ML, et al. A tunica vaginalis testis tumor in a 20 year old man. Ann Pathol 2000;20:633–4.
6. Xiao SU, Rizzo P, Carbone M. Benign papillary mesothelioma of the tunica vaginalis. Arch Pathol Lab Med 2000;124:143–7.
7. Goldblum J, Hart WR. Localized and diffuse mesotheliomas of the genital tract and peritoneum in women: a clinicopathologic study of nineteen true mesothelial neoplasms, other than adenomatoid tumors, multicystic mesotheliomas and localized fibrous tumors. Am J Surg Pathol 1995;19:1124–37.

8. Yesner R, Hurtwitz A. Localized pleural mesothelioma of epithelial type. J Thorac Surg 1953;26:325–9.
9. Butnor K, Sporn TA, Hammar SP, et al. Well-differentiated papillary mesothelioma. Am J Surg Pathol 2001;25:1304–9.
10. Galateau-Salle F, Vignaud JM, Burke L, et al. Well differentiated papillary mesothelioma of the pleura: a series of 24 cases. Am J Surg Pathol 2004: 28:534–40.
11. Daya D, Mc Caughey WTE. Pathology of the peritoneum: a review of selected topics. Semin Diagn Pathol 1991;8:277–89.
12. Clement PB, Young RH, Scully RE. Malignant mesotheliomas presenting as ovarian masses. Am J Surg Pathol 1996;20:1067–80.
13. Truong LD, Maccato ML, Awat H, et al. Serous surface carcinoma of the peritoneum: a clinicopathologic study of 22 cases. Hum Pathol 1990;21:99–110.
14. Jones MA, Young RH, Scully RE. Malignant mesothelioma of the tunica vaginalis: a clinicopathologic analysis of 11 cases with review of the literature. Am J Surg Pathol 1995;19:815–25.
15. Katsube Y, Mukai K, Silverberg SG. Cystic mesothelioma of the peritoneum: a report of five cases and review of the literature. Cancer 1982;50:1615–22.
16. Weiss SW, Tavassoli FA. Multicystic mesothelioma: an analysis of pathologic findings and biologic behavior in 37 cases. Am J Surg Pathol 1988;12:737–46.
17. Goldblum J, Hart WR. Localized and diffuse mesotheliomas of the genital tract and peritoneum in women: a clinicopathologic study of nineteen true mesothelial neoplasms, other than adenomatoid tumors, multicystic mesotheliomas, and localized fibrous tumors. Am J Surg Pathol 1995;19:1124–37.
18. Lamovec J, Sinkovec J. Multilocular peritoneal inclusion cyst (multicystic mesothelioma) with hyaline globules. Histopathology 1996;28:466–9.
19. Drut R, Quijano G. Multilocular mesothelial inclusion cysts (so-called benign multicystic mesothelioma) of pericardium. Histopathology 1999;34:472–4.
20. Ball NJ, Urbanski SJ, Green FH, et al. Pleural multicystic mesothelial proliferation: the so-called muticystic mesothelioma. Am J Surg Pathol 1990;14:375–8.
21. Scucchi L, Mingazzini P, Di Stefano D, et al. Two cases of "multicystic peritoneal mesothelioma": description and critical review of the literature. Anticancer Res 1994;14:715–20.
22. Attanoos RL, Gibbs AR. Pathology of malignant mesothelioma. Histopathology 1997;30:403–18.
23. Niggli FK, Gray TJ, Raafat F, et al. Spectrum of peritoneal mesothelioma in childhood: clinical and histopathologic features, including DNA cytometry. Pediatr Hematol Oncol 1994;11:399–408.
24. Mutafoglu-Uysal K, Kargi A, Sarialioglu F, et al. Malignant pleural mesothelioma in a child: long-term survival with ICE-WAC chemotherapy regimen. Turk J Pediatr 2002;44:244–7.
25. Candanedo-Gonzalez F, Luna-Perez P. [Cystic lymphangioma of the mesentery: clinical, radiological, and morphological analysis.] Rev Gastroenterol Mex 2000; 65:6–10.
26. Heatley MK, Russell P. Florid cystic endosalpingiosis of the uterus. J Clin Pathol 2001;54:399–400.

11 Differential Diagnosis: Nonmesothelial Lesions

Reactive Squamous Metaplasia

Reactive squamous metaplasia is a rare event with reactive and malignant mesothelial lesions of the pleura (Figure 11.1) [1]. Squamous metaplasia may rarely be seen on the pleura of patients with cystic fibrosis. The main pitfall in diagnosis is with metastatic well-differentiated squamous cell carcinoma from adjacent viscera or from extension of a microscopic peripheral pulmonary squamous cell carcinoma. In the absence of squamous pearls, bladder carcinoma metastatic to the pleura has to be considered in the differential diagnosis.

Nodular Histiocytic Mesothelial Hyperplasia

Nodular histiocytic/mesothelial hyperplasia is a rare tumor-like lesion first described by Rosai and Dehner in 1975 in hernial sacs [2]. It is characterized by nodules distributed at the surface of the pleura and composed almost exclusively of large histiocytic cells showing a mild degree of atypia and round to oval nuclei (Figure 11.2) [3, 4]. The bland cytology of the lesion associated with the strong reactivity for CD68 and the absence of cytokeratin positivity, except for some scattered reactive mesothelial cells, indicate the correct diagnosis. Because histiocytes/macrophages exhibit CD31 positivity, this lesion could also be mistaken for epithelioid hemangioendothelioma [4]. Nodular histiocytic mesothelial hyperplasia appears to be identical to mesothelial/monocytic incidental cardiac excrescences [5], which probably result from irritation to the mesothelial lining by various causes leading to focal aggregation of histiocytes in the serosal cavity. The clues to recognizing the true nature of the lesion are clinicopathologic correlation and identification of CD68-positive/cytokeratin-negative cells. Similarly, displaced mesothelial cells in the visceral pleura do not appear to penetrate beyond the pleural elastic lamina or into the subjacent lung parenchyma.

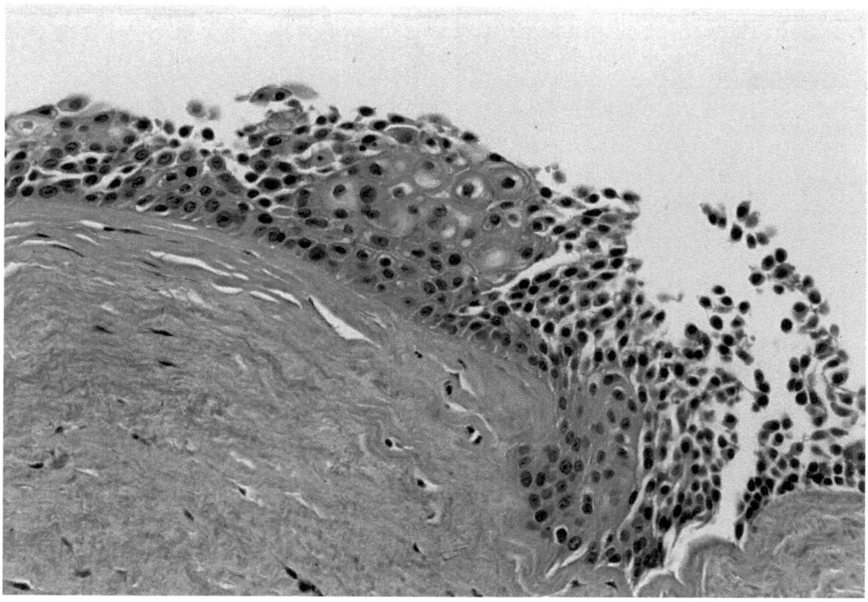

FIGURE 11.1. Reactive squamous metaplasia in the pleura.

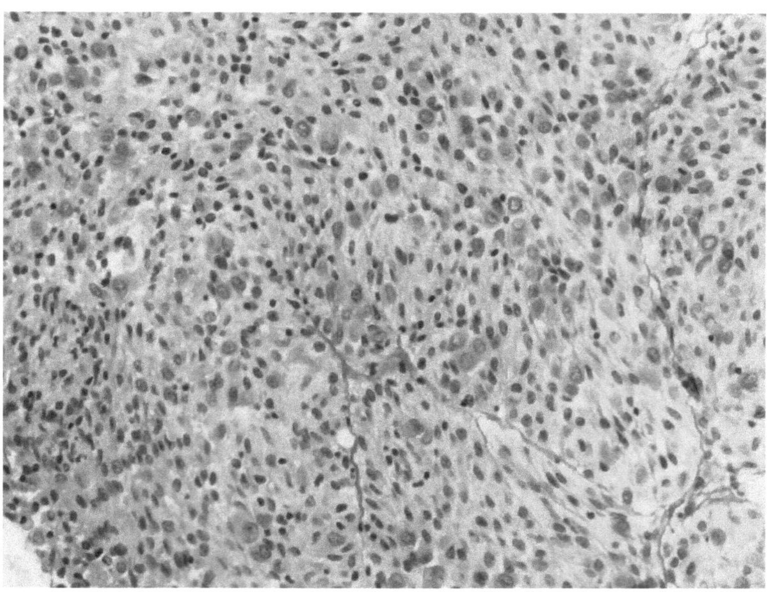

A

FIGURE 11.2. A. Pleural nodular histiocytic hyperplasia mimicking malignant mesothelioma. B. Same case: CD 68 immunopositivity. C. Same case calretirin immunopositivity.

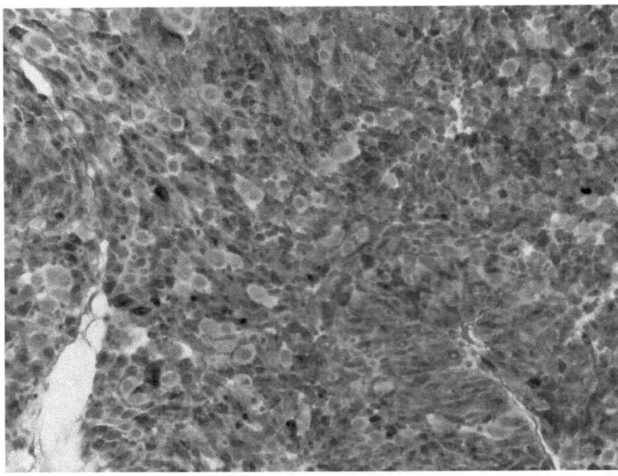

B

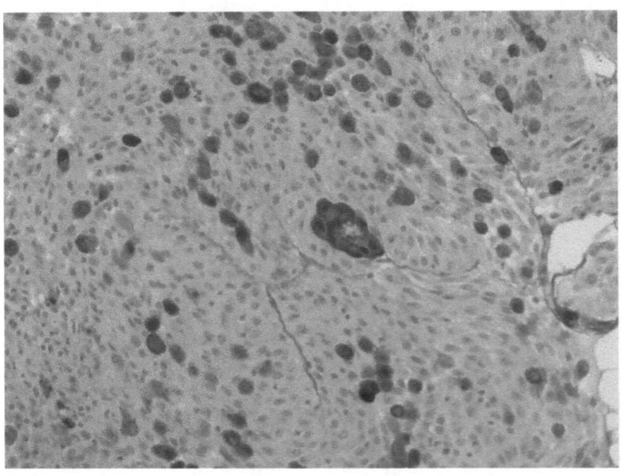

C

FIGURE 11.2. *Continued*

Endosalpingiosis and Endometriosis

Endosalpingiosis and endometriosis may involve the peritoneum and have the potential to be confused with mesothelioma. An important distinguishing feature is the presence of columnar cells sometimes ciliated and frequently associated with hemorrhage. As a rule, endosalpingiosis and endometriosis are focal processes [6].

Ectopic Decidua

Ectopic decidua (Figure 11.3) is a common finding in young women. It should not to be confused with deciduoid malignant mesothelioma as the

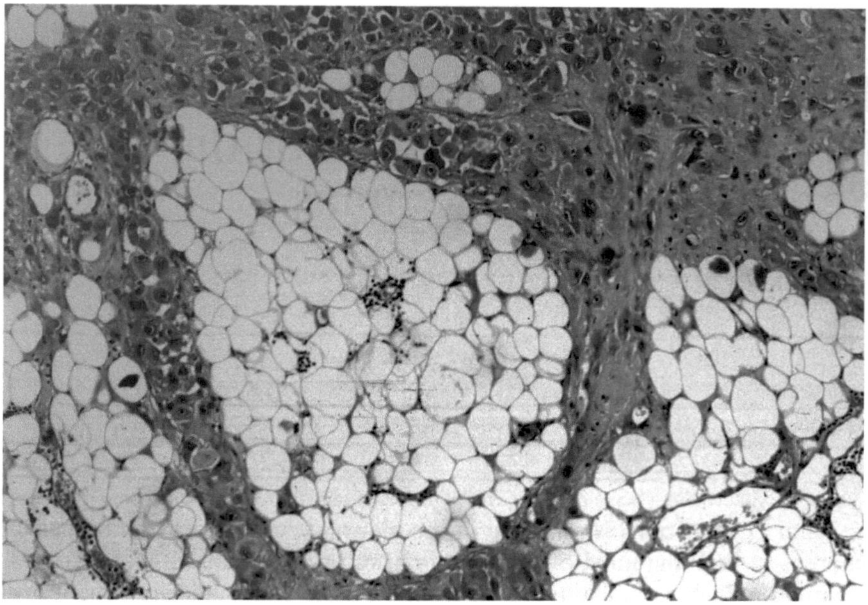

FIGURE 11.3. Florid deciduoid change in the peritoneum 6 months after pregnancy. There is no invasion of adipose tissue.

latter shows estrogen receptor and progesterone receptor negativity and calretinin positivity.

References

1. Willen R, Bruce T, Dahlstrom G, et al. Squamous epithelial cancer in metaplastic pleura following extrapleural pneumothorax for pulmonary tuberculosis. Virchows Arch A Pathol Anat Histol 1976;370:225–31.
2. Rosai J, Dehner LP. Nodular mesothelial hyperplasia in hernia sacs: a benign reactive condition simulating a neoplastic process. Cancer 1975;35:165–75.
3. Chan JKC, Loo KT, Yau BKC, et al. Nodular histiocytic/mesothelial hyperplasia: a lesion potentially mistaken for a neoplasm in transbronchial biopsy. Am J Surg Pathol 1997;21:658–63.
4. Ordonez NG, Ayala AG. Lesions described as nodular mesothelial hyperplasia are primarily composed of histiocytes. Am J Surg Pathol 1998;22:285–92.
5. Luthringer DJ, Virmani R, Weiss SW, et al. A distinctive cardiovascular lesion resembling histiocytoid (epithelioid) hemangioma: evidence suggesting mesothelial participation. Am J Surg Pathol 1990;14:993–1000.
6. Vilos GA, Vilos AW, Haebe JJ. Laparoscopic findings, management, histopathology, and outcome of 25 women with cyclic leg pain. J Am Assoc Gynecol Laparosc 2002;9:145–51.

12 Differential Diagnosis: Nonmesothelial Tumors of the Serosal Cavity: Sarcomas

Synovial Sarcoma

Synovial sarcomas (SSs) consist of biphasic and monophasic types (Figures 12.1 and 12.2). Most SSs reported in the pleural cavity have been biphasic, whereas in the lung most of the tumors have been monophasic [1, 2].

Biphasic SS can be distinguished from biphasic malignant mesothelioma (MM) by the following criteria. Biphasic SS occurs at a younger age (mean 25 years; range 9–50 years) than MM (mean age 65 years; range 40–80 years) [1, 3]. Biphasic SS is usually localized although diffuse lesions may be seen, whereas MM causes diffuse pleural thickening. Histologically, SSs show long, interweaving fascicles, frequent hemangiopericytomatous pattern, and hyaline fibrosis. In contrast, MM rarely shows long fascicles and rarely displays a hemangiopericytomatous pattern. Moreover, in SS the nuclei demonstrate finely dispersed chromatin and inconspicuous nucleoli, whereas small central nucleoli and margination of the chromatin are seen in MM. Biphasic SS typically shows positive mucin staining, whereas this feature is usually negative in mesotheliomas. In most cases of SS, carcinoembryonic antigen (CEA) expression is seen in the glandular element, whereas it is only rarely seen in epithelioid mesotheliomas. S100 may be positive in SS, but it is usually negative in mesothelioma. SS frequently express bcl2, in contrast to mesotheliomas. Biphasic SS shows large geographic areas of membranous and cytoplasmic staining for epithelial membrane antigen (EMA) (Figure 12.3). Epithelioid mesotheliomas typically show cell membrane positivity for EMA. Calretinin is expressed by both mesotheliomas and synovial sarcomas. By electon microscopy, synovial sarcomas are seen to have short, blunt microvilli whereas MMs have long, bushy microvilli [4, 5]. The t(X,18) translocation is seen in SS but is not observed in MM [6].

Monophasic SS [6] potentially can occur in the pleural cavity but would be very difficult to distinguish from sarcomatoid malignant mesothelioma. Favoring the diagnosis of a monophasic SS would be a localized, rather than diffuse, macroscopic distribution and histologic features of long,

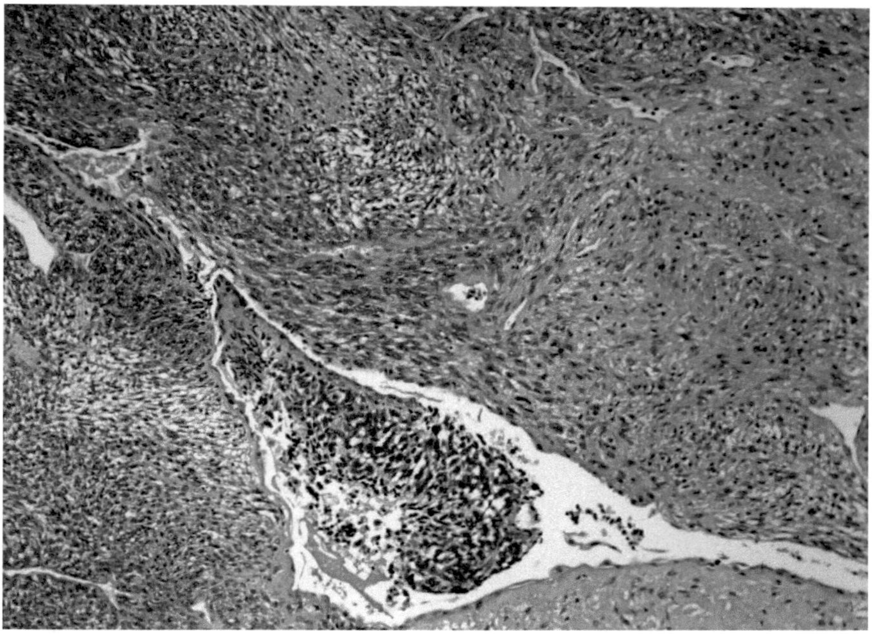

FIGURE 12.1. Monophasic synovial sarcoma, showing small dark cells and relatively paucicellular myxoid areas.

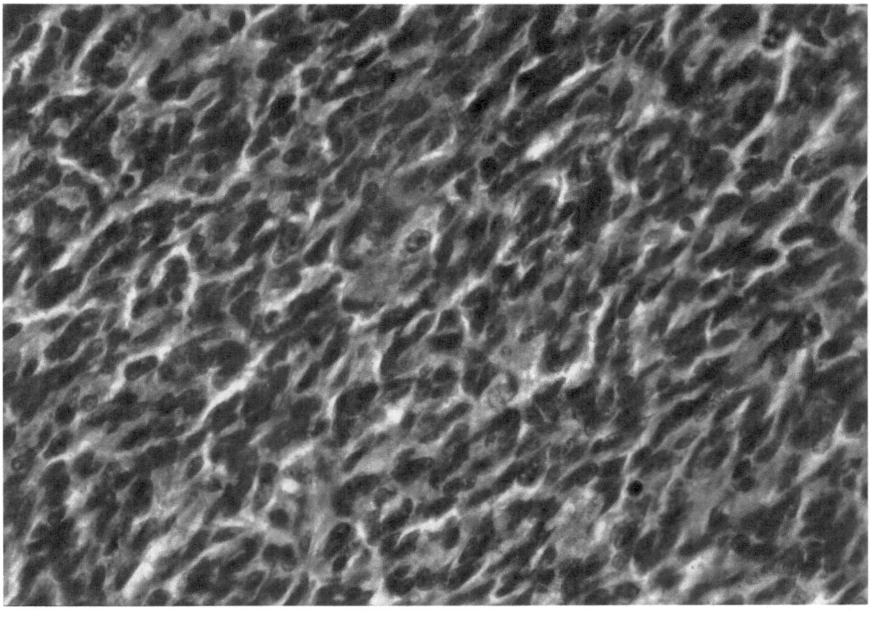

FIGURE 12.2. Monophasic synovial sarcoma, showing fascicles of dark spindle cells.

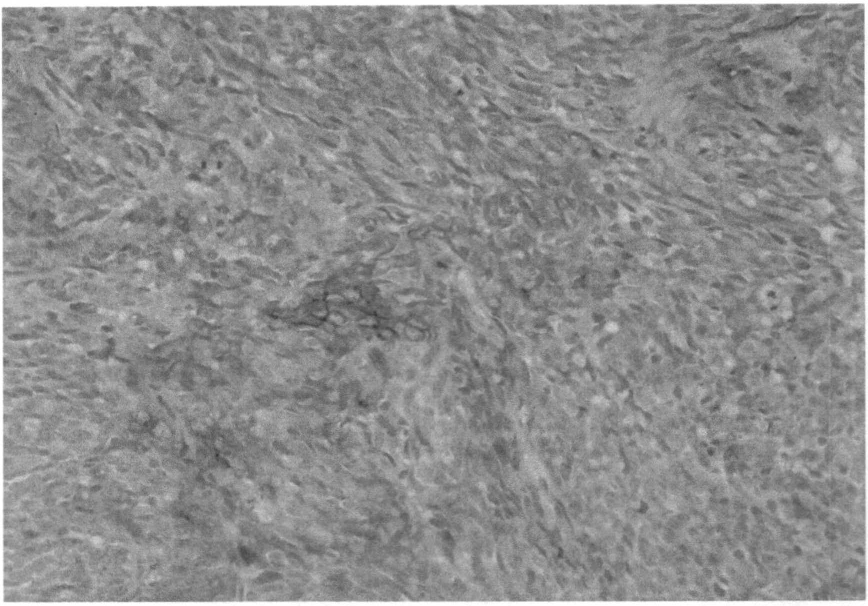

FIGURE 12.3. Synovial sarcoma, showing focal membranous epithelial membrane antigen (EMA) immunostaining.

interweaving fascicles and frequently a hemangiopericytomatous pattern. Immunohistochemistry for CEA and electron microscopy are usually not helpful owing to lack of a glandular component. It has been suggested that positive bcl2 may favor SS, as its presence in mesothelioma appears to be infrequent [6–8]. Identification of the t(X:18) translocation indicates SS [8].

Poorly differentiated SS (PDSS) is characterized by a highly cellular proliferation made up of large rounded cells with numerous mitoses and necrosis, and it may be observed in the pleura. PDSS may be overlooked in this location because it may be extremely difficult to differentiate PDSS from poorly differentiated mesothelioma in the absence of molecular cytogenetics analysis for t(x:18) (SYT-SSX) as they usually have the same immunohistochemical profile as malignant mesothelioma [1, 7].

Epithelioid Hemangioendothelioma and Angiosarcoma

Malignant epithelioid vascular tumors presenting in the pleura embrace a spectrum of lesions, from low grade epithelioid hemangioendotheliomas [9] to high grade angiosarcomas [10, 11]. Epithelioid hemangioendotheliomas are composed of short cords and nests of epithelioid endothelial cells frequently embedded in a myxohyaline matrix. The tumor cells have sharply defined cytoplasmic vacuoles and frequently exhibit a vascular growth pattern and hyaline necrosis (Figures 12.4–12.6]. The cytoplasmic vacuoles represent intracytoplasmic lumens within which red blood cells may be seen. Abortive vessel formation is a helpful morphologic clue to vascular differentiation. The intermixture of epithelioid cells and fibroblastic stroma may give a biphasic appearance that mimics biphasic malignant mesothelioma. Epithelioid vascular tumors may show higher degrees of cytologic atypia, forming an epithelioid angiosarcoma [11].

Epithelioid hemangioendothelioma or angiosarcoma may present with diffuse pleural thickening but more often these lesions present in the lung as multiple nodules. Some patients have pulmonary nodules and pleural involvement. Epithelioid hemangioendothelioma and angiosarcoma can occur in a variety of other sites as well, such as the liver, soft tissue, and bone; they and may present in multiple organs simultaneously. The prognosis is poor, with death in less than 1 year regardless of whether the tumor is an epithelioid hemangioendothelioma or an angiosarcoma [9, 10, 11, 12]. There is no clear association with asbestos exposure [9].

Immunohistochemistry in most cases is positive for vascular markers, including CD31, CD34, and factor VIII [10, 12]. These tumors can be difficult to diagnose because occasionally the neoplastic cells express keratin, suggesting a mesothelioma or carcinoma. Staining for vimentin is usually

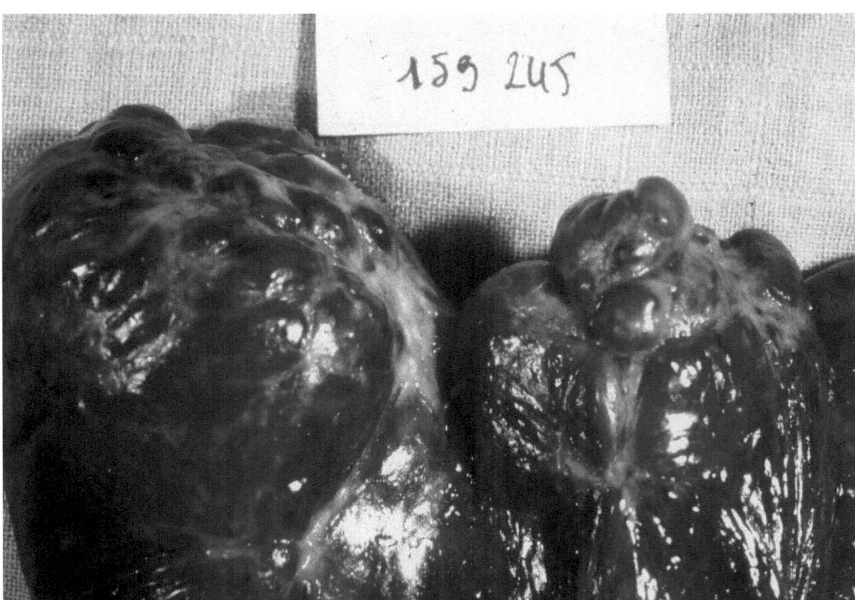

FIGURE 12.4. Epithelioid hemangioendothelioma, showing "net-like" external compression of lung.

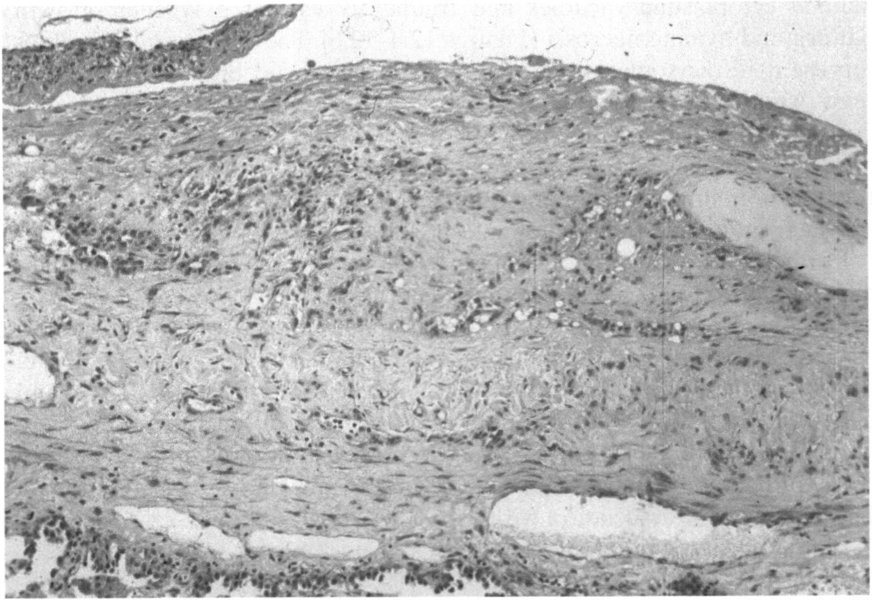

FIGURE 12.5. Epithelioid hemangioendothelioma, showing typical epithelioid cells set in a myxoid fibrous stroma.

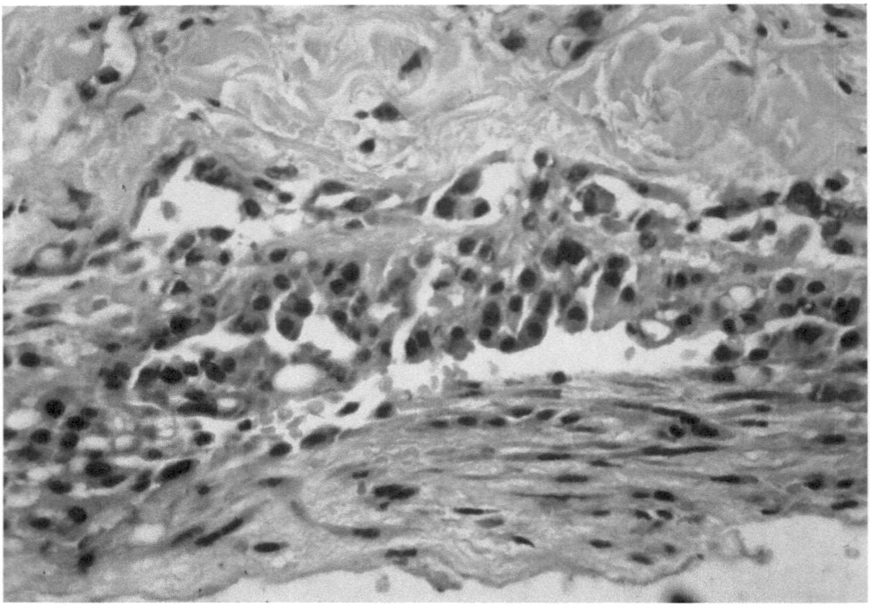

FIGURE 12.6. Epithelioid hemangioendothelioma, showing typical epithelioid cells with intracellular lumen filled with red blood cells.

strongly positive [10–12]. Calretinin is typically negative. Unless one considers the diagnosis, the correct immunohistochemical studies and ultrastructural evaluation are not done. In some of the cases, Wiebel-Palade bodies are seen in the cytoplasm of these cells and are pathognomonic markers of endothelial cells. This neoplasm often has a poor prognosis.

Leiomyosarcoma

Leiomyosarcomas may occur in the pleura as metastatic or primary neoplasms and are composed of fascicles of eosinophilic spindle cells with ovoid, vesicular, to cigar-shaped nuclei. They usually demonstrate positivity for smooth muscle actin, desmin, or both [13]. About 30% to 40% of leiomyosarcomas at all locations are immunopositive for cytokeratins and EMA, making the differential diagnosis with sarcomatoid mesotheliomas extremely difficult. Some sarcomatoid mesotheliomas show smooth muscle differentiation with expression of actin, desmin, keratin, and vimentin; [14] and they have ultrastructural features of myoid or myofibroblastic differentiation.

Benign and Malignant Peripheral Nerve Sheath Tumor

Both benign and malignant peripheral nerve sheath tumor can occur in the pleural cavity. When benign they typically have such morphologic features as Antoni A and B areas, hyaline vascular changes, and Verocay bodies. Neurofibromas demonstrate interlacing bundles of elongated cells with wavy nuclei within a wire-like collagen and mucoid matrix. When malignant they may lack these features and mimic malignant solitary fibrous tumor and sarcomatoid mesothelioma as well. Positive staining with S-100 is helpful for confirming a neurogenic origin [11, 14].

Primitive Neuroectodermal Tumor

Primitive neuroectodermal tumors (PNETs) consist of sheets of discohesive, small, round tumor cells with frequent areas of necrosis [16]. PNET and Ewing's sarcoma represent a spectrum of small round cell sarcoma that for the purposes of this discussion is called PNET. Rosette-like structures are common, and cystic spaces may be formed. There is a high nuclear/cytoplasmic ratio, and the nuclei typically have vesicular or finely granular chromatin (Figure 12.7). Nucleoli may be present. Glycogen can often be demonstrated in the cytoplasm utilizing periodic acid-Schiff (PAS) stain with and without diastase. Immunohistochemistry characteristically is positive for MIC2 [15, 16] and negative for keratin. However, focal positivity

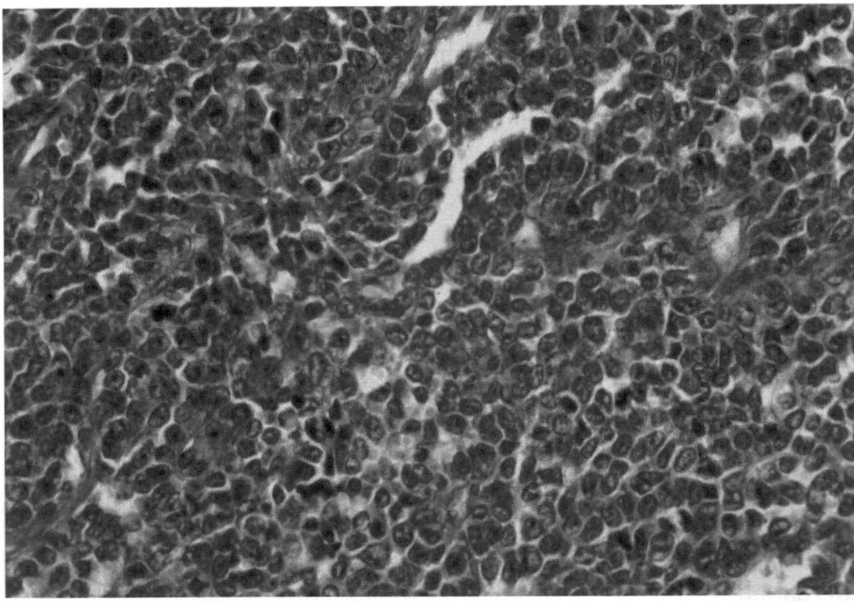

FIGURE 12.7. Primitive neuroectodermal tumor ("Askin tumor") showing sheets of dark round cells.

can be seen for keratin, chromogranin, or synaptophysin. Histologically, these tumors could be confused with small cell mesotheliomas.

The tumors tend to be large, localized masses when involving the pleural cavity; and they usually also extend into the chest wall, lung parenchyma, or both. They tend to occur in children and young adults. Rarely, they are confused with malignant mesothelioma because of their presentation as a pleural mass; their morphologic features are more likely to be confused with small cell carcinoma, lymphoma, or other small round blue cell tumors. Molecular analysis reveals a characteristic translocation: t(11;22)(q24;q12) although this is not specific [16]. Molecular studies and immunohistochemistry must be interpreted in the context of appropriate histologic features [16, 17, 18].

Desmoid Tumor

Desmoid tumors are rarely pleural [19]. They often present clinically as large masses with a mean diameter of 12.5 cm (range 5–16 cm). They may involve either the parietal or visceral pleura and usually have a sessile attachment without a pedicle. Histologically, they consist of intersecting fascicles of bland spindled fibroblastic cells interspersed with a loose fibrillar collagenous matrix and focal, dense, laminated collagen, reminiscent of a

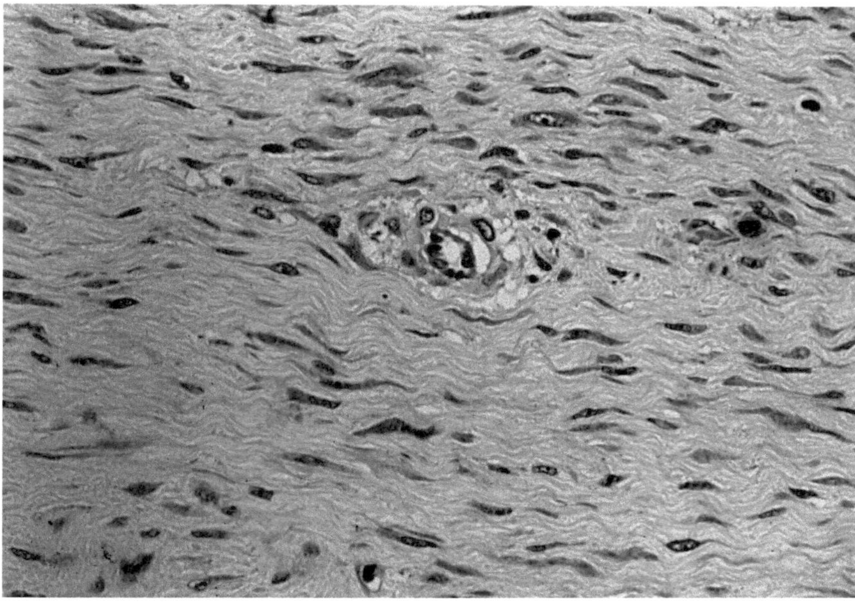

FIGURE 12.8. Desmoid tumor showing cells with elongated, wavy nuclei.

localized fibrous tumor. The tumor cells are thin with wavy to elongated nuclei that have sharp, pointed ends (Figure 12.8). The tumors are infiltrative, growing into surrounding soft tissues. Mitoses, pleomorphism, and necrosis are absent.

Immunohistochemistry may be positive for vimentin, smooth muscle actin, muscle-specific actin, and desmin. However, CD34, S-100 protein, and cytokeratin are negative [19]. These tumors must be separated from localized fibrous tumors and neurogenic tumors. Localized fibrous tumors tend to show a distinctive stromal ropy collagen that is uncommon in desmoid tumors, which are more likely to show a loose fibrillar collagenous matrix.

Desmoplastic Round Cell Tumor

Desmoplastic round cell tumor is a malignant lesion composed of nests of small round cells in a dense fibrous or cellular spindle-celled stroma. This tumor presents most often in the abdomen or pelvis [20], although cases have been reported rarely in the pleura [21, 22], thorax [23], and paratesticular region [24]. Most patients are adolescents or young adults [20]. The tumor cells usually have scant cytoplasm and some nuclear molding (Figure 12.9). Immunohistochemically, they are typically positive for cytokeratin and desmin, often with a dot-like cytoplasmic pattern. Immunohistochemistry for WT1 is also typically positive, in contrast to PNETs [25, 26].

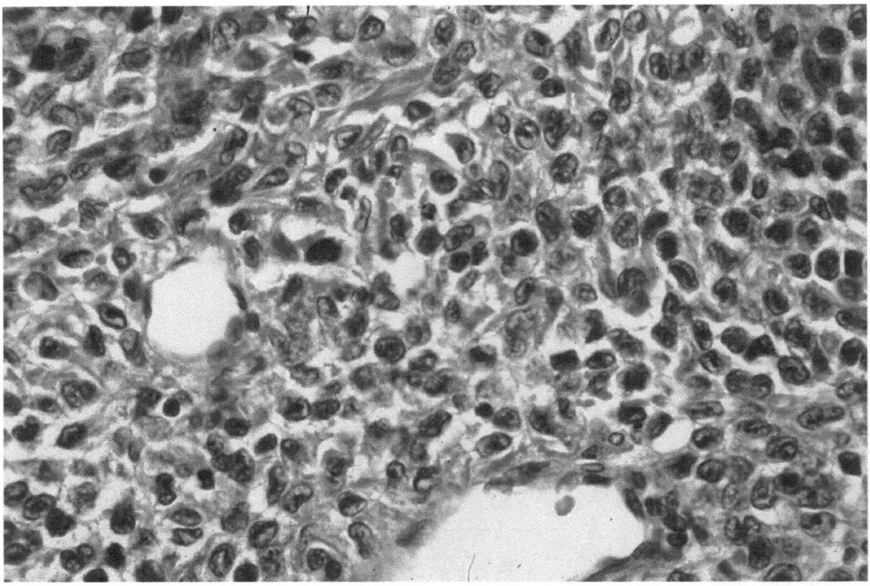

FIGURE 12.9. Desmoplastic round cell tumor with focal collagenization.

These tumors are characteristically found to have the translocation t(11;22)(p13;q12) by molecular analysis [27].

Pleuropulmonary Blastoma

Pleuropulmonary blastoma is a cystic or solid neoplasm (or both) in which the cystic component is lined by benign metaplastic epithelium that may be ciliated [28, 29]. When these neoplams are exclusively cystic, the malignant component consists of primitive small cells underneath the epithelium with a cambium layer-like appearance, as is seen in sarcoma botryoides. Focal rhabdomyoblasts may be found among the malignant small cells (Figure 12.10). Solid areas have differentiated or anaplastic sarcomatous elements (or both) including embryonal rhabdomyosarcoma, fibrosarcoma, chondrosarcoma, anaplastic undifferentiated sarcoma, and mixtures of these cell types [30]. Solid islands of primitive cells separated by a myxoid spindle cell stroma may resemble the blastema in Wilms' tumor.

Pleuropulmonary blastoma is a dysontogenic malignant neoplasm of early childhood that may involve the lung or pleura (or both). Cystic pleuropulmonary blastoma may mimic benign cystic lung disease and hamartomatous lesions. There is a family history of similar-appearing intrathoracic tumors, other solid tumors of childhood, and various malformations in up to 30% of cases. This tumor must be distinguished from pulmonary

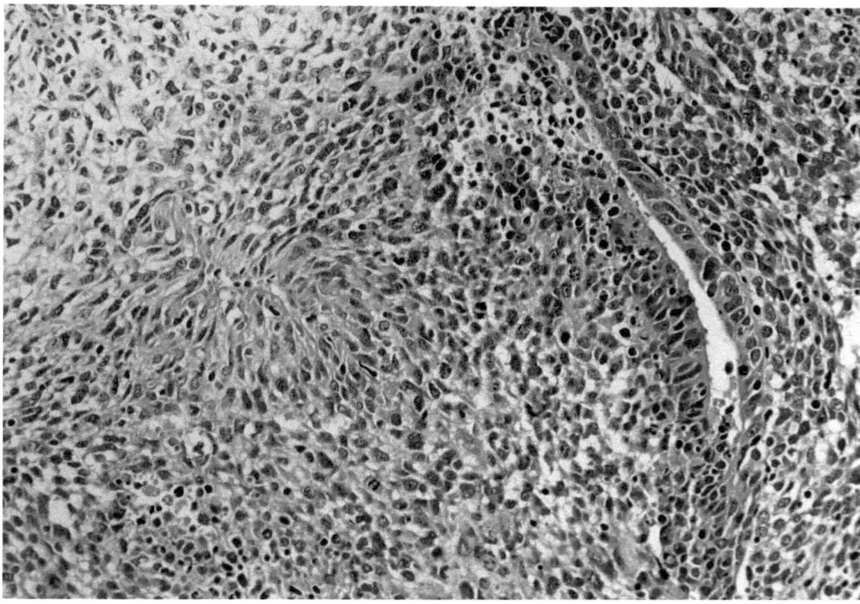

FIGURE 12.10. Pleuropulmonary blastoma showing.

blastoma, which characteristically occurs in adults. A favorable prognosis correlates with the extent of cystic change [29].

Inflammatory Myofibroblastic Tumor

Inflammatory pseudotumor shows a spectrum of fibroblastic or myofibroblastic proliferations with a varying infiltrate of inflammatory cells, typically plasma cells, lymphocytes, and foamy histiocytes. The lesions may range from a primarily myofibroblastic or fibroxanthomatous appearance to one that has a heavy infiltrate of plasma cells. These tumors usually occur in the lung, and rarely they involve the pleura. Whether they represent a reactive or a neoplastic lesion is not known. They can show invasive growth and, if not completely excised, may recur. Other terms that have been used for this tumor include inflammatory myofibroblastic tumor, plasma cell granuloma, fibroxanthoma, fibrous histiocytoma, and pseudosarcomatous myoblastic tumor.

Other sarcomas can rarely occur in the pleura, including liposarcoma [30], rhabdomyosarcoma [31], and others that have already been discussed [14].

References

1. Gaertner E, Zeren H, Fleming MV, et al. Biphasic synovial sarcomas arising in the pleural cavity: a clinicopathologic study of five cases. Am J Surg Pathol 1996;20:36–45.
2. Kaplan MA, Goodman MD, Satish J, et al. Primary pulmonary sarcoma with morphologic features of monophasic synovial sarcoma and chromosome translocation t(X;18). Am J Clin Pathol 1996;105:195–9.
3. Nicholson AG, Goldstraw P, Fisher C. Synovial sarcoma or the pleura and its differentiation from other primary pleural tumours: a clinicopathological and immunohistochemical review of three cases. Histopathology 1998;33:508–13.
4. Jawahar DA, Vuletin JC, Gorecki P, et al. Primary biphasic synovial sarcoma of the pleura. Respir Med 1997;91:568–70.
5. Zeren H, Moran CA, Suster S, et al. Primary pulmonary sarcomas with features of monophasic synovial sarcoma: a clinicopathological, immunohistochemical, and ultrastructural study of 25 cases. Hum Pathol 1995;26:474–80.
6. De Leeuw B, Suijkerbuijk RF, Olde Weghuis D, et al. Distinct Xp 11.2 breakpoint regions in synovial sarcoma revealed by metaphase and interphase FISH: relationship to histologic subtypes. Cancer Genet Cytogenet 1994;73:89–94.
7. Begueret H, Galateau-Salle F, Guillou L, et al. Primary intrathoracic synovial sarcoma. A clinicopathologic study of 40 t(x: 18)-positive cases from the French sarcoma group and Mesopath group. Am J Surg Pathol 2005;29:339–46.
8. Guillou L, Benhattar J, Bonichon F, et al. Histologic grade, but not SYT-SSX fusion type, is an important prognostic factor in patients with synosial sarcoma: a multicenter, retrospective analysis. J Clin Oncol 2004;22:4040–50.
9. Attanoos RL, Suvarna SK, Rhead E, et al. Malignant vascular tumour in "asbestos" workers and endothelial differentiation in malignant mesothelioma. Thorax 2000;55:860–3.
10. Lin BT, Colby T, Gown AM, et al. Malignant vascular tumors of the serous membranes mimicking mesothelioma: a report of 14 cases. Am J Surg Pathol 1996;20:1431–9.
11. Fletcher C, Krishnan Unni K, Mertens F. Tumour of soft tissue and bone. Lyon: WHO IARC Press; 2002.
12. Zhang PJ, Livolsi VA, Brooks JJ. Malignant epithelioid vascular tumors of the pleura: report of a series and literature review. Hum Pathol 2000;31:29–34.
13. Mayall FG, Goddard H, Gibbs AR. "Intermediate filament" expression in mesotheliomas: leiomyoid mesotheliomas are not "uncommon." Histopathology 1992;21:453–7.
14. Ordonez NG, Tornos C. Malignant peripheral nerve sheath tumor of the pleura with epithelial and rhabdomyoblastic differentiation: report of a case clinically simulating mesothelioma. Am J Surg Pathol 1997;21:1515–21.
15. Dehner LP. Primitive neuroectodermal tumor and Ewing's sarcoma. Am J Surg Pathol 1993;17:1–13.
16. Perlman EJ, Dickman PS, Askin FB, et al. Ewing's sarcoma—routine diagnostic utilization of MIC2 analysis: a Pediatric Oncology Group/Children's Cancer Group Intergroup Study. Hum Pathol 1994;25:304–7.
17. Weidner N, Tjoe J. Immunohistochemical profile of monoclonal antibody O13: antibody that recognizes glycoprotein p30/32MIC2 and is useful in diagnosing

Ewing's sarcoma and peripheral neuroepithelioma. Am J Surg Pathol 1994; 18:486–94.
18. Thorner P, Squire J, Chilton-MacNeil S, et al. Is the EWS/FLI-1 fusion transcript specific for Ewing sarcoma and peripheral primitive neuroectodermal tumor? A report of four cases showing this transcript in a wider range of tumor types. Am J Pathol 1996;148:1125–38.
19. Wilson RW, Galateau-Salle F, Moran CA. Desmoid tumors of the pleura: a clinicopathologic mimic of localized fibrous trumor. Mod Pathol 1999;12:9–14.
20. Schwarz RE, Gerald WL, Kushner BH, et al. Desmoplastic small round cell tumors: prognostic indicators and results of surgical management. Ann Surg Oncol 1998;5:416–22.
21. Parkash V, Gerald WL, Parma A, et al. Desmoplastic small round cell tumor of the pleura. Am J Surg Pathol 1995;19:659–65.
22. Sapi Z, Szentirmay Z, Orosz Z. Desmoplastic small round cell tumour of the pleura: a case report with further cytogenetic and ultrastructural evidence of "mesothelioblastemic" origin. Eur J Surg Oncol 1999;25:633–4.
23. Venkateswaran L, Jenkins JJ, Kaste SC, et al. Disseminated intrathoracic desmoplastic small round-cell tumor: a case report. J Pediatr Hematol Oncol 1997;19:172–5.
24. Cummings OW, Ulbright TM, Young RH, et al. Desmoplastic small round cell tumors of the paratesticular region: a report of six cases. Am J Surg Pathol 1997;21:219–25.
25. Barnoud R, Sabourin JC, Pasquier D, et al. Immunohistochemical expression of WT1 by desmoplastic small round cell tumor: a comparative study with other small round cell tumors. Am J Surg Pathol 2000;25:830–6.
26. Hill DA, Pfeifer JD, Marley EF, et al. WT1 staining reliably differentiates desmoplastic small round cell tumor from Ewing sarcoma/primitive neuroectodermal tumor: an immunohistochemical and moleculardiagnostic study. Am J Clin Pathol 2000;114:345–53.
27. Liu J, Nau MM, Yeh JC, et al. Molecular heterogeneity and function of EWS-WT1 fusion transcripts in desmoplastic small round cell tumors. Clin Cancer Res 2000;6:3522–9.
28. Manivel JC, Priest JR, Watterson J, et al. Pleuropulmonary blastoma: the so-called pulmonary blastoma of childhood. Cancer 1988;62:1516–26.
29. Priest JR, McDermott MB, Bhatia S, et al. Pleuropulmonary blastoma: a clinicopathologic study of 50 cases. Cancer 1997;80:147–61.
30. Okby NT, Travais WD. Liposarcoma of the pleural cavity. Arch Pathol Lab Mad 2000;124:699–703.
31. Hamada T, Tanimoto A, Kaido M, et al. Diffuse pleural rhabdomyosarcoma with persistent pleural effusion. Acta Pathol Jpn 1989;39:803–9.

13
Differential Diagnosis: Other Nonmesothelial Tumors

Solitary Fibrous Tumor

Solitary fibrous tumors are uncommon. They can arise from the serous membranes and many other locations, such as lung parenchyma, upper respiratory tract, mediastinum, and orbit [1–4]. In the serous cavities they are thought to develop from fibroblasts of the submesothelial connective tissue [5].

They are usually solid but can be cystic and often have a pedicle (Figure 13.1). There is no convincing association with asbestos exposure. Both benign (most of the tumors) and malignant forms can occur, although the behavior of individual tumors is difficult to predict.

They vary in cellularity, with densely packed spindle and oval-shaped cells to acellular collagenous areas. They show a variety of patterns, including haphazardly arranged interlacing fascicles ("patternless"), herringbone, "hemangiopericytoma-like," neural-like, diffuse sclerosing, and loose myxoid (Figures 13.2 and 13.3). These tumors can show calcification. Features suggesting a malignant or more aggressive behavior [1, 6] are (1) >4 mitoses per 10 high power fields; (2) the presence of abnormal mitotic figures; (3) cellular pleomorphism; (4) the presence of tumor giant cells; (5) size larger than 10 cm; (6) areas of necrosis; (7) prominent nucleoli; (8) lack of a pedicle. Disseminated solitary fibrous tumor may occur [7].

Solitary fibrous tumors usually do not stain immunohistochemically for cytokeratin, S100, or desmin but are positive for vimentin and focally for SMA. CD34 is a useful positive marker for LFT but is not specific [3]. The neoplastic cells are diffusely positive for bcl2 and CD99 [8]. CD34 does not usually stain mesotheliomas. However, the malignant forms of localized fibrous tumors may fail to stain immunohistochemically for CD34 [8] and a small proportion of sarcomatoid mesotheliomas are negative for cytokeratin [9].

When the tumor is benign, well localized, and has a pedicle, there should be no difficulty distinguishing it from malignant mesothelioma. However,

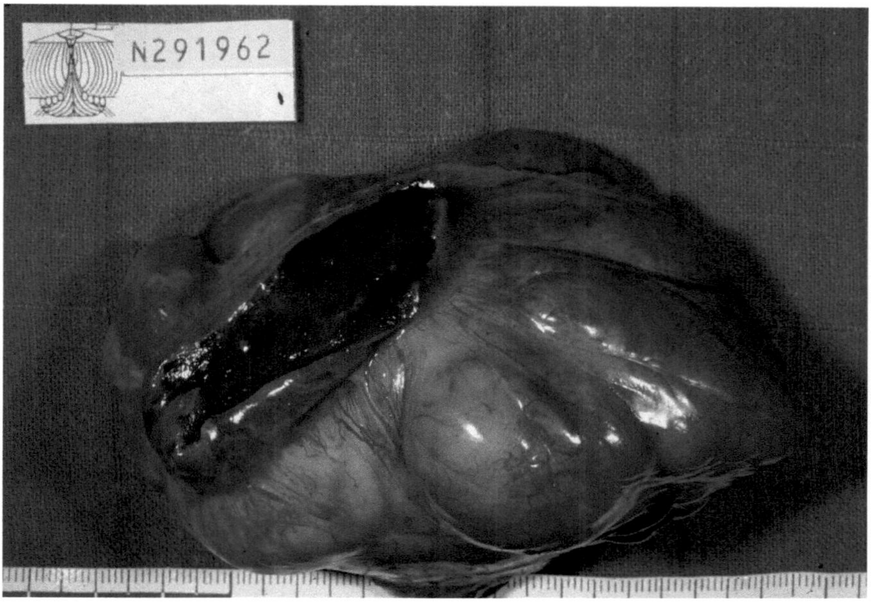

FIGURE 13.1. Solitary fibrous tumor with a pedicle.

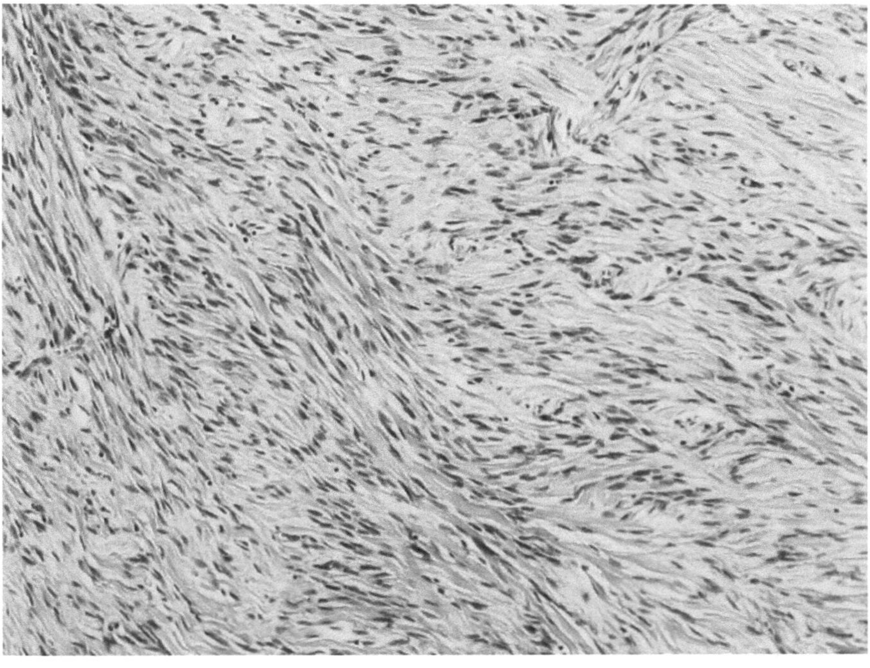

FIGURE 13.2. Solitary fibrous tumor, showing the patternless and hemangiopericytic pattern.

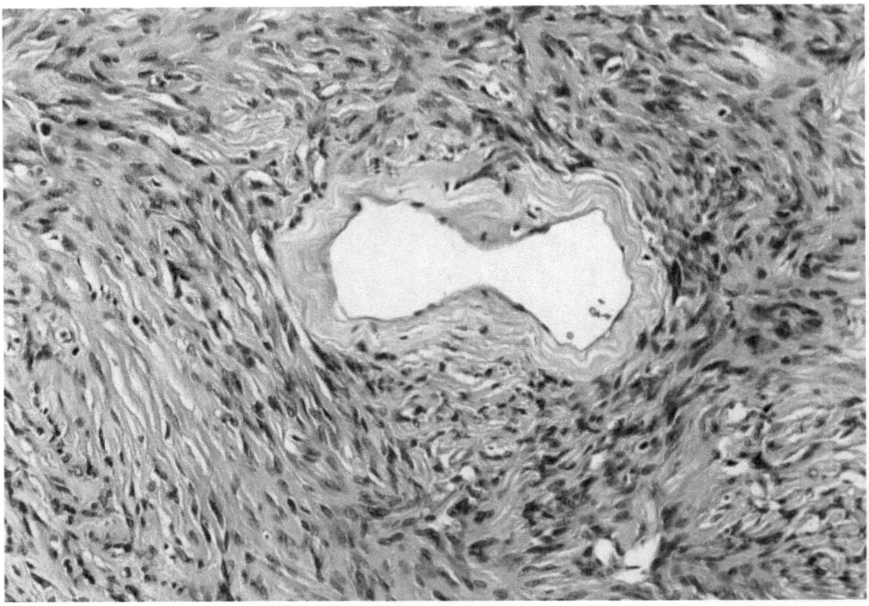

FIGURE 13.3. Same case, high power view as a vessel.

when it is large and toward the malignant end of the spectrum, it may be difficult to differentiate from the sarcomatoid forms of malignant mesothelioma.

Calcifying Fibrous Pseudotumor

Calcifying fibrous pseudotumor rarely presents in the pleura or peritoneum [10–12]. It appears as solitary lesions in young adults. It also may present as multiple serosal masses or plaque-like lesions [12]. Calcifying fibrous pseudotumor has some clinical and pathologic features in common with inflammatory myofibroblastic tumors and may recur locally, but it has not been reported to metastasize [13]. It is characterized by densely hyalinized or laminated collagen with few spindle cells and calcification with either psammomatous or dystrophic features (Figure 13.4). In some cases there is a lamellar appearance to the calcifications. Chronic inflammation consisting of lymphocytes and plasma cells is mild. Calcifying fibrous pseudotumor of the pleura is distinct from calcified granulomas, calcified pleural plaques, and chronic fibrous pleuritis as well as other calcifying intrapulmonary lesions such as hyalinizing granuloma, inflammatory pseudotumor, and amyloid. The pathogenesis of the lesion is still unclear [14].

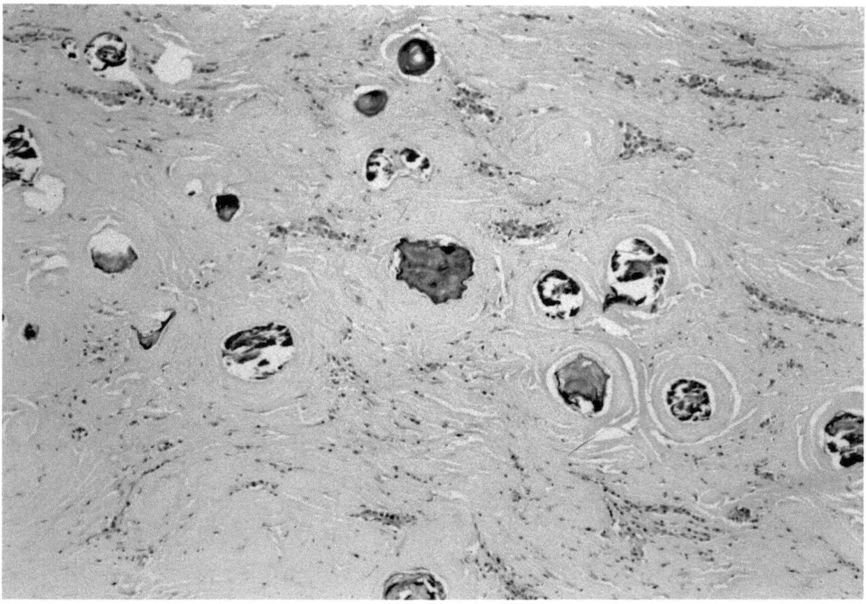

FIGURE 13.4. Calcifying fibrous pseudotumor with hyalinized collagen and numerous round, laminated, calcified structures.

Leiomyomatosis Peritonealis Disseminata

Leiomyomatosis peritonealis disseminata is defined by the presence of multiple peritoneal nodules composed of plump fusiform cells that resemble smooth muscle cells. It is usually an incidental finding during the course of laparoscopy or laparotomy for postpartum tubal ligation or during cesarean section. It is mostly seen in women of reproductive age and during pregnancy, although it may occur in oral contraceptive users (70%). It can occur in postmenopausal women. Leiomyomatosis is considered to be the result of metaplastic transformation of suberosal mesenchymal cells and may be observed in the vicinity of ectopic decidua, endosalpingiosis, and endometriosis [15]. Caution should be used when interpreting these lesions in pregnant or postpartum women as the cells may have the intermediate appearance of decidual cells and smooth muscle and may be misdiagnosed as a malignant deciduoid mesothelioma when the lesion is particularly florid [16]. The calretinin negativity of cells and the absence of definite invasion of adipocytes should prevent a false diagnosis of deciduoid or sarcomatoid mesothelioma.

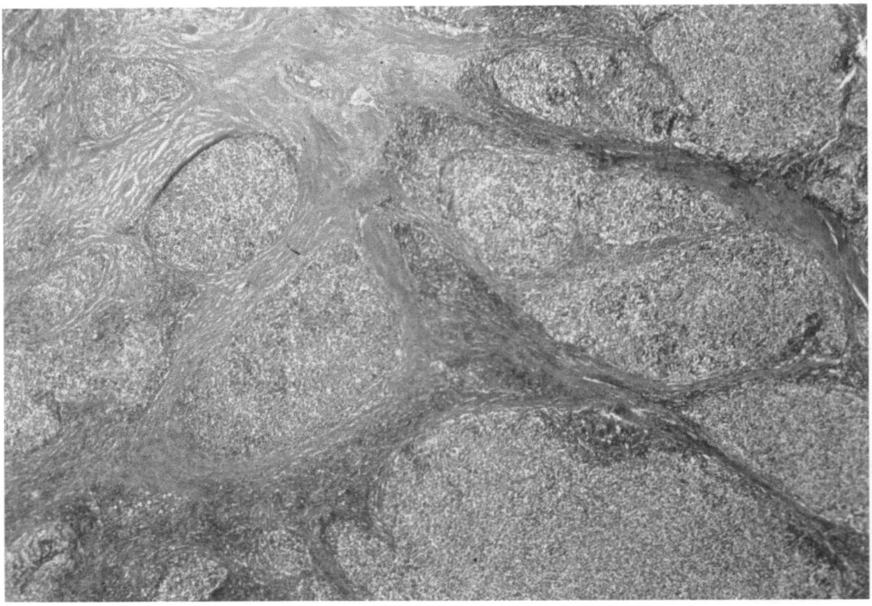

FIGURE 13.5. Intrapulmonary thymoma showing typical lobulation.

Thymoma/Thymic Carcinoma

Thymic tumors arise rarely in the pleura and may form localized or diffuse masses, the latter mimicking malignant mesothelioma. Moran et al. [17] and Attanoos et al. [18] have each reported eight cases. Light microscopically, the tumors can simulate epithelioid, biphasic, sarcomatoid, and lymphohistiocytic forms of mesothelioma. Important clues to the diagnosis include a prominent lobulated architecture and perivascular edema (Figure 13.5) containing lymphocytes of T-cell phenotype, neither of which is seen in mesothelioma. Attanoos et al. [18] demonstrated that intrapleural thymic tumors may express the mesothelioma markers (CK5/6) (8/8), calretinin (8/8), and thrombomodulin (1/8). Calretinin was expressed only in stromal cells. Nuclear expression was not seen in the thymic epithelial cells. The lymphoid component in types B1, B2, and B3 commonly shared an immune phenotype with expression of CD1a, CD2, CD99, and TdT. The presence of an immature T-cell phenotype in an epithelial malignancy strongly suggests a diagnosis of thymic epithelial tumor.

Melanoma

Malignant melanomas can spread to the pleura, producing a pseudomesotheliomatous appearance. They can exhibit a variety of light microscopic patterns, including large and small epithelial cell, spindle cell, and pleomorphic patterns. Therefore light microscopically, melanoma may potentially mimic epithelioid, sarcomatoid, and biphasic malignant mesothelioma.

S100 and HMB45 are useful markers for melanoma. S100 is more sensitive but less specific than HMB45; 10% to 15% of melanomas are negative for HMB45 [19]; 20% of melanomas are positive for low-molecular-weight cytokeratins, particularly the desmoplastic spindle cell form [20]. Electron microscopy may be useful for the differential diagnosis by showing the presence of melanosomes in melanoma or long, slender microvilli in mesothelioma.

Serous Carcinoma

Serous carcinoma can arise from the ovary and peritoneum of women (secondary müllerian system) and when disseminated can be difficult to distinguish from diffuse malignant peritoneal mesothelioma, particularly when there is a prominent papillary architecture [21–24] Histologic features, such as the degree of nuclear atypia, stratification, and tufting, may be helpful but are of limited use (Figure 13.6). Psammoma bodies can occur in serous carcinomas and mesotheliomas. Similarly, direct stains for neutral mucin such as periodic acid-Schiff (PAS)–diastase are of little value because a high proportion of serous carcinomas do not show positive staining. There is a paucity of studies comparing the immunohistochemical profile of epithelioid peritoneal mesothelioma with serous carcinomas of the peritoneum and ovary [25]. Epithelial markers, such as carcinoembryonic antigen (CEA), are not useful, being negative in both mesothelioma and serous carcinoma. The most useful diagnostic panel appears to be calretinin and CK5/6, which are frequently positive (88% and 53%, respectively) in epithelioid peritoneal mesothelioma and usually negative in the serous carcinomas (0% and 25%, respectively), and BerEP4 appeared to be the most useful epithelial marker, being positive in 95% of serous carcinomas and 9% of mesotheliomas [25].

Lymphomas of the Serosal Cavities

Lymphomas of the serosal cavities are being addressed in the WHO 2004 classification of lung, pleural, thymic, and cardiac tumors; and therefore the classification given below may be superceded.

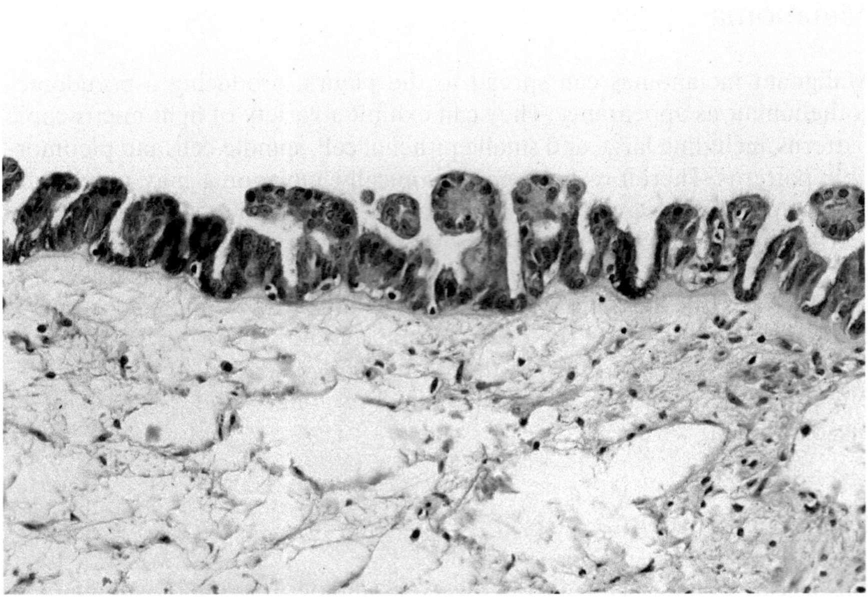

FIGURE 13.6. Serous carcinoma, showing epithelial stratification and tufting. Note the rare cilia at the top of occasional cells.

Lymphomatous involvement of the pleura is most commonly due to systemic stage IV disease and theoretically can occur from any of the recognized Revisited European American Lymphoma [REAL] classification entities. Primary pleural lymphomas are rare and the most frequently recognized REAL/WHO entities at this site are body cavity (serous effusion)-based lymphomas and pyothorax-associated lymphoma. *Body cavity (effusion)-based lymphomas*, which are associated with human immunodeficiency virus (HIV) infection, frequently present with effusions in serous cavities. They do not usually produce clinically apparent masses but, instead, comprise large blastic and mitotically active lymphoid cells in suspension (Figure 13.7) [26, 27]. They are usually positive for CD20, CD30, and CD79a and may be negative for CD45. HHV8 and Epstein-Barr virus (EBV) are usually presentas seen by the polymerase chain reaction (PCR) or Southern blot analysis (Figure 13.8) [28, 29, 30].

Pyothorax-associated lymphomas have been described mostly in East Asians in association with long-standing (more than 20 years typically) chronic inflammation of the pleural cavity, such as pyothorax or tuberculous pleuritis [29, 30]. They are not associated with HIV infection. They are composed of large blastic lymphoid cells with immunoblastic morphology. They are usually CD45- and CD20-positive but negative for epithelial membrane antigen (EMA). They are positive for EBV and negative for HHV8 [31–32].

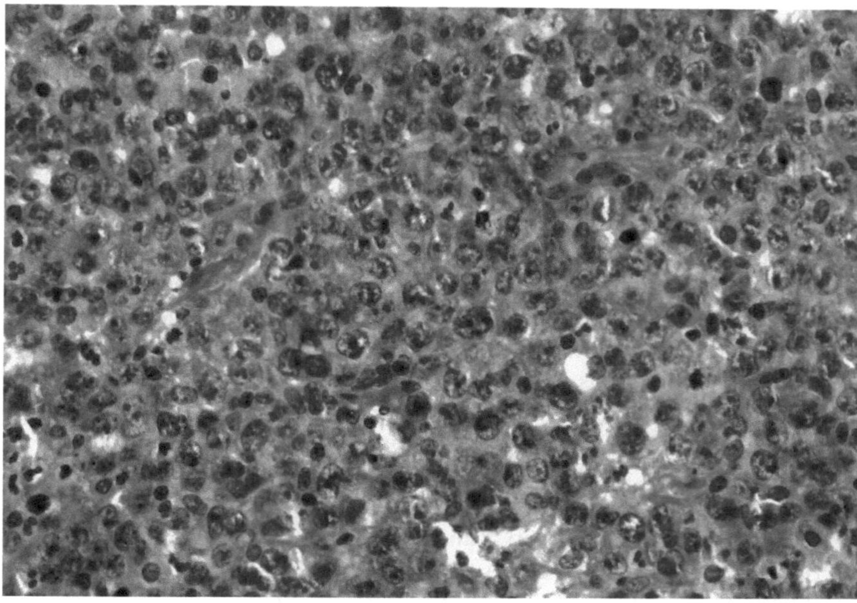

FIGURE 13.7. High grade malignant BALT lymphoma occurring as a body cavity (effusion)-based lymphoma.

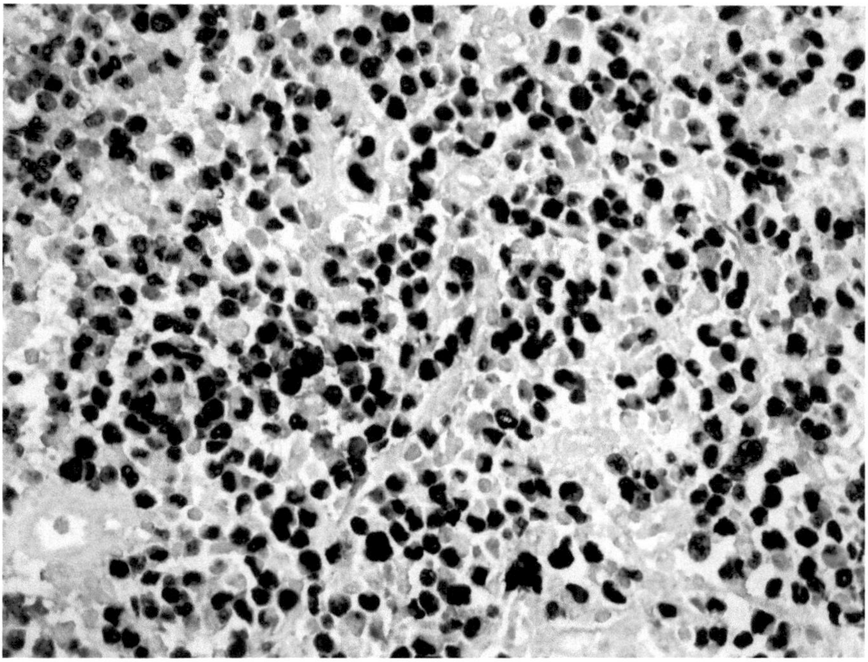

FIGURE 13.8. Same case, showing Epstein-Barr virus nuclear positivity by in situ hybridization.

Other Lymphomas That May Involve the Pleura

Diffuse large B-cell lymphoma represents the largest single category in the REAL/WHO classification, comprising approximately 30% of all non-Hodgkin lymphomas. Pleuropulmonary involvement has been described rarely in the absence of nodal or marrow involvement. By light microscopy, the tumor is seen to be composed of sheets of large blastic cells, some of which may show an immunoblastic morphology with plasmatocytoid basophilic cytoplasm and large nuclei with a central prominent nucleolus. An anaplastic morphology may also be seen where the tumor cells show more abundant cytoplasm and there is considerable nuclear atypia with multinucleate giant cells. Mitoses are frequent (atypical forms in the anaplastic cases), and the proliferation marker Ki-67 reveals 20% to 90% cycling cells. Immunophenotypically, all patients express CD45 and are of B-cell phenotype (CD20- and CD79a-positive). Extranodal cases often express bcl-2 and bcl-6 oncoproteins. Small reactive T cells (CD3-positive) are present in variable numbers. Tumors showing prominent plasmacytoid differentiation may express EMA. Anaplastic morphology is usually associated with expression of the activation marker CD30.

Primary sclerosing mediastinal B-cell lymphoma often presents in young Females with superior vena caval obstruction, and pleuropulmonary involvement may occur. The tumor is thought to arise from mature thymic B lymphocytes. The blastic lymphoid cells may have multilobated or cleaved nuclear profiles with clear cell cytoplasm and are intimately associated with a lobular delicate fibrosis. The tumor immunotype comprises CD45, CD20, and CD30 positivity. CD15 is negative, allowing distinction from Hodgkin's lymphoma.

Anaplastic large cell lymphomas can spread to the pleura to mimic mesothelioma. They are highly anaplastic tumors wilth large round, oval, or polygonal cells with bizarre pleomorphic nuclei. They are difficult to distinguish from carcinoma, melanoma, sarcoma, and mesothelioma. They can be misdiagnosed because they are sometimes CD45-negative, and half show EMA positivity. Almost all stain for CD30 and occasionally CD15. A high proportion of the EMA-positive patients express the t2:5 translocation associated with ALK-1 chimeric protein production; these lesions represent a good prognostic group. They may rarely be CAM5.2-positive.

Rarely, nonhematopoietic tissues, including mesothelium, may express CD30 [33]. Awareness of this possibility is important to prevent misdiagnosis.

References

1. England DM, Hochholzer L, McCarthy MJ. Localised benign and malignant fibrous tumour of the pleura. Am J Surg Pathol 1989;13:640–58.
2. Briselli M, Mark EJ, Dickersin GR. Solitary fibrous tumour of the pleura: eight new cases and review of 360 cases in the literature. Cancer 1981;47:2678–89.

3. Flint A, Weiss SW. CD-34 and keratin expression distinguishes solitary fibrous tumour (fibrous mesothelioma) of pleura from desmoplastic mesothelioma. Hum Pathol 1995;26:428–31.
4. Khalifa MA, Montgomery EA, Azumi N, et al. Solitary fibrous lesions: a series of lesions, some in unusual sites. South Med J 1997;90:793–9.
5. Bolen JW. Tumors of serosal origin. Clin Lab Med 1987;7:31–50.
6. Moran CA, Suster S, Koss MN. The spectrum of histologic growth patterns in benign and malignant fibrous tumour of the pleura. Semin Diagn Pathol 1992; 9:169–80.
7. Zhang H, Lucas DR, Pass HI, et al. Disseminated malignant solitary fibrous tumor of the pleura. Pathol Int 2004;54:111–5.
8. Yokoi T, Tsuzuki M, Yatabe Y, et al. Solitary fibrous tumor: significance of p53 and CD34 immunoreactivity in its malignant transformation. Histopathology 1998;32:423–32.
9. Cavazza A, Rossi G, Agostini L, et al. Cytokeratin-positive malignant solitary fibrous tumour of the pleura: an unusual pitfall in the diagnosis of pleural spindle cell neoplasms. Histopathology 2003;43:606–8.
10. Hainaut P, Lesage V, Weynand B, et al. Calcifying fibrous pseudotumor (CFPT): a patient presenting with multiple pleural lesions. Acta Clin Belg 1999;54: 162–4.
11. Pinkard NB, Wilson RW, Lawless N, et al. Calcifying fibrous pseudotumor of pleura: a report of three cases of a newly described entity involving the pleura. Am J Clin Pathol 1996;105:189–94.
12. Fetsch JF, Montgomery EA, Meis JM. Calcifying fibrous pseudotumor. Am J Surg Pathol 199317:502–8.
13. Van Dorpe J, Ectors N, Geboes K, et al. Is calcifying fibrous pseudotumor a late sclerosing stage of inflammatory myofibroblastic tumor? Am J Surg Pathol 1999;23:329–35.
14. Kocova L, Michal M, Sulc M, et al. Calcifying fibrous pseudotumour of visceral peritoneum. Histopathology 1997;31:182–4.
15. Vilos GA, Vilosan Haebe JJ. Leiomyomatosis peritonealis disseminated endometriosis and multicystic mesothelioma: an unusual association. Int J Gynecol Pathol 1998;17:178–82.
16. Zotalis G, Nayar R, Hicks DG. Leiomyomatosis peritonealis disseminata, endometriosis, and multicystic mesothelioma: an unusual association. Int J Gynecol Pathol 1998;17:178–82.
17. Moran CA, Travis WD, Rosado-de-Christenson M, et al. Thymomas presenting as pleural tumour. Am J Surg Pathol 1992;16:138–44.
18. Attanoos RL, Galateau-Salle F, Gibbs AR, et al. Primary thymic epithelial tumour of the pleura mimicking malignant mesothelioma. Histopathology 2002; 41:42–9.
19. Jungbluth AA, Busam KJ, Gerald WL, et al. An anti-melanoma monoclonal antibody for the detection of malignant melanoma in parffin embedded tissues. Am J Surg Pathol 1998;22:595–602.
20. Zarbo RJ, Gowan AM, Nagle RB, et al. Anomalous cyokeratin expression in malignant melanoma: one-and-two-dimensional Western blot analysis and immunohistochemical survery of 100 melanomas. Mod Pathol 1990;3: 494–501.

21. Bollinger DJ, Wick MR, Dehner LP, et al. Peritoneal malignant mesothelioma vs serous papillary adenocarcinoma: a histochemical and immunohistochemical comparison. Am J Surg Pathol 1989;13:659–70.
22. Foyle A, Al-Jabi M, McCaughey WTE, et al. Papillary peritoneal tumour in women. Am J Surg Pathol 1981;5:241–9.
23. Kannerstein M, Churg J, McCaughey WTE, et al. Papillary tumour of the peritoneum in women: mesothelioma or papillary carcinoma. Am J Obstet Gynecol 1977;127:306–14.
24. Raju U, Fine J, Greenwald KA, et al. Primary papillary serous neoplasia of the peritoneum: a clinicopathologic and ultrastructural study of 8 cases. Hum Pathol 1989;20:426–36.
25. Webb R, Attanoos RL, Dojcinov SD, et al. Value of mesothelial and epithelial antibodies in distinguishing diffuse peritoneal mesothelioma in females from serous papillary carcinoma of the ovary and peritoneum. Histopathology 2002; 40:237–44.
26. Ansari MQ, Dawson DB, Nador R, et al. Primary body cavity-based AIDS-related lymphomas. Am J Clin Pathol 1996;105:221–9.
27. Jaffe ES. Primary body cavity-based AIDS-related lymphomas. Am J Clin Pathol 1996;105:141–2.
28. Cesarman E, Chang Y, Moore PS, et al. Kaposi's sarcoma-associated herpesvirus-like DNA sequences in AIDS-related body-cavity-based lymphomas. N Engl J Med 1995;332:1186–91.
29. Iuchi K, Aozasa K, Yamoto S, et al. Non-Hodgkin's lymphomas of the pleural cavity developing from long-standing pyothorax. Jpn J Clin Oncol 1989;19: 249–57.
30. Martin A, Capron F, Liguory-Brunaud M, et al. Epstein-Barr-virus-associated primary malignant lymphomas of the pleural cavity occurring in long standing pleural chronic inflammation. Hum Pathol 1994;25:1314–8.
31. Fukayama M, Ibuka T, Hayashi Y, et al. Epstein-Barr virus in pyothorax-associated pleural lymphoma. Am J Pathol 1993;143:1044–9.
32. Bryant-Greenwood P, Sorbara L, Filie AC, et al. Infection of mesothelial cells with human herpes virus 8 in human immunodeficiency virus-infected patients with Kaposi's sarcoma, Castleman's disease, and recurrent pleural effusions. Mod Pathol 2003;16:145–53.
33. Dunphy CH, Gardner LJ, Bee CS. Malignant mesothelioma with CD30 positivity. A case report and review of the laterature. Arch Pathol Lab Med 2000;124:1077–9.

Appendix

Appendix 1. WHO International Histologic Classification of Tumors, Fourth Edition, 2004.

- Diffuse malignant mesothelioma
  - Epithelioid mesothelioma
  - Sarcomatoid mesothelioma
  - Desmoplastic mesothelioma
  - Biphasic mesothelioma
- Other tumors of mesothelial origin
  - Well-differentiated papillary mesothelioma
  - Adenomatoid tumor
- Lymphoproliferative disorders
  - Primary effusion lymphoma
  - Pyothorax-associated lymphoma
- Mesenchymal tumors
  - Epithelioid hemangioendothelioma
    - Angiosarcoma
  - Synovial sarcoma
    - Monophasic
    - Biphasic
  - Solitary fibrous tumor
  - Calcifying tumor of the pleura
  - Desmoplastic round cell tumor of the pleura

Appendix 2. WHO Histologic Classification of Tumors of the Peritoneum (Lyon: IARC, 2003).

- Peritoneal tumors
- Mesothelial tumors
  - Diffuse malignant mesothelioma
  - Well-differentiated papillary mesothelioma
  - Multicystic mesothelioma
  - Adenomatoid tumor
- Smooth muscle tumor
  - Leiomyomatosis peritonealis disseminate
- Tumor of uncertain origin
  - Desmoplastic round cell tumor
- Epithelial tumors
  - Primary peritoneal serous adenocarcinoma
  - Primary peritoneal borderline tumor (specify type)
  - Others

APPENDIX 3. International Staging System for Malignant Pleural Mesothelioma.

TNM Clinical Classification

T	Primary tumor
Tx	Primary tumor cannot be assessed
T0	No evidence of primary tumor
T1	
T1a	Tumor limited to the ipsilateral parietal pleura, including mediastinal and diaphragmatic pleura. No involvement of the visceral pleura
T1b	Tumor involving the ipsilateral parietal pleura including mediastinal and diaphragmatic pleura. Scattered foci of tumor also involving the visceral pleura
T2	Tumor involving each of the ipsilateral pleural surfaces (parietal mediastinal diaphragmatic and visceral pleura) with at least one of the following features:
	Involvement of diaphragmatic muscle
	Confluent visceral pleural tumor (including the fissues) or extension of tumor from visceral pleura into the underlying pulmonary parenchyma
T3	Describes locally advanced but potentially resectable tumor
	Tumor involving all of the ipsilateral pleural surfaces (parietal, mediastinal, diaphragmatic, and visceral pleura) with at least one of the following features:
	Involvement of the endothoracic fascia
	Extension into the mediastinal fat
	Solitary, completely resectable focus of tumor extending into the soft tissues of the chest wall
	Nontransmural involvement of the pericardium
T4	Locally advanced, technically unresectable tumor
	Tumor involving all of the ipsilateral pleural surfaces (parietal, mediastinal, diaphragmatic, and visceral) with at least one of the following features:
	Diffuse extension or multifocal masses of tumor in the chest wall, with or without associated rib destruction
	Direct transdiaphragmatic extension of tumor to the peritoneum
	Direct extension of tumor to the contralateral pleura
	Direct extension of tumor to one or more mediastinal organs
	Direct extension of tumor into the spine
	Tumor extending through to the internal surface of the pericardium with or without a pericardial effusion; or tumor involving the myocardium
N	Lymph nodes
Nx	Regional lymph nodes cannot be assessed
N0	No regional lymph node metastases
N1	Metastases in the ipsilateral bronchopulmonary or hilar lymph nodes
N2	Metastases in the subcarinal or the ipsilateral mediastinal lymph nodes, including the ipsilateral internal mammary nodes
N3	Metastases in the contralateral mediastinal, contralateral internal mammary, ipsilateral, or contralateral supraclavicular lymph nodes
M -	Metastases
Mx	Presence of distant metastases cannot be assessed
M0	No distant metastasis
M1	Distant metastasis present

Stage

Stage I	Ia	T1aN0M0
	1b	T1bN0M0
Stage II		T2N0M0
Stage III		Any T3M0
		Any N1M0
		Any N2M0
Stage IV		Any T4
		Any N3
		Any M1

Rusch VW. A proposed new international TNM staging system for malignant pleural mesothelioma from the international mesothelioma interest group. Lung Cancer 1996;14:1–12.

Appendix 4. TNM Classification

Rules for Classification According to the WHO

The classification applies only to malignant mesothelioma of the pleura. There should be histologic confirmation of the disease. The following are the procedures for assessing T, N, and M categories.

T categories: physical examination, imaging, endoscopy, and/or surgical exploration
N categories: physical examination, imaging endoscopy, and/or surgical examination
M categories:physical examination, imaging endoscopy, and/or surgical examination

Regional Lymph Nodes

The regional lymph nodes are the intrathoracic, scalene, and supraclavicular nodes.

TNM Clinical Classification

T—Primary Tumor

TX	Primary tumor cannot be assessed
T0	No evidence of primary tumor
T1	Tumor limited to ipsilateral parietal and/or visceral pleura
T2	Tumor invades any of the following: ipsilateral lung, endothoracic fascia, diaphragm, pericardium
T3	Tumor invades any of the following: ipsilateral chest wall muscle, ribs, mediastinal organs or tissues
T4	Tumor directly extends to any of the following: contralateral pleura, contralateral lung, peritoneum, intraabdominal organs, cervical tissues

N—Regional Lymph Nodes

Nx	Regional lymph nodes cannot be assessed
N0	No regional lymph node metastasis
N1	Metastasis in ipsilateral peribronchial and/or ipsilateral hilar lymph nodes, including involvment by direct extension
N2	Metastasis in ipsilateral mediastinal and/or subcarinal lymph node(s)
N3	Metastasis in contralateral mediastinal, contralateral hilar, ipsilateral or contralateral scalene, or supraventricular lymph node(s)

M—Distant Metastasis

Mx	Distant metastasis cannot be assessed
M0	No distant metastasis
M1	Distant metastasis

pTNM Pathologic Classification

The pT, pN, and pM categories correspond to the T, N, and M categories.

Stage Grouping

Stage I	T1N0M0
	T2N0M0
Stage II	T1N1M0
	T2N1M0
Stage III	T1N2M0
	T2N2M0
	T3N0/N1/N2M0
Stage IV	Any TN3M0
	T4Any NM0
	Any TAny NM1

Appendix 5. Specimen Reporting

Patient name
Date of surgery
Date of receipt of specimen
Site
Type of specimen
Report of frozen section diagnosis
Frozen material available (yes/no)*Time from surgery to arrival in the laboratory*

Clinical history: type of pleural involvement, localized or diffuse, any intrapulmonary involvement, history of previous malignancy

Histologic diagnosis
- Specify as listed above
- Comment about any uncertainty (see diagnostic terminology below)
- If lung parenchyma is present: assess for other lesions, including asbestos bodies (iron stains)

Immunohistochemistry results: summarize (if done) in comment
Electron microscopy results: summarize (if done) in comment

Index

Note: Page numbers followed by f indicate figures: t indicates tables.

MIX
Papier aus verantwortungsvollen Quellen
Paper from responsible sources
FSC® C105338

If you have any concerns about our products,
you can contact us on
ProductSafety@springernature.com

In case Publisher is established outside the EU,
the EU authorized representative is:
Springer Nature Customer Service Center GmbH
Europaplatz 3, 69115 Heidelberg, Germany

Printed by Libri Plureos GmbH
in Hamburg, Germany